THE SPACES IN BETWEEN

A Journeying into Self Evolution

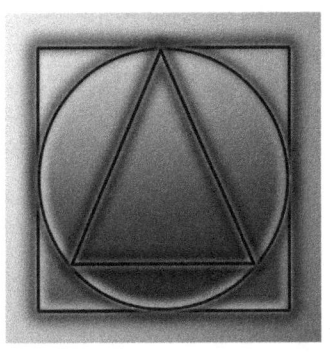

GEOFF HUNNEF

The Spaces in Between
Copyright © 2020 by Geoff Hunnef

All rights reserved. No part of this publication
may be reproduced, distributed, or transmitted
in any form or by any means, including
photocopying, recording, or other electronic
or mechanical methods, without the prior
written permission of the author, except
in the case of brief quotations embodied
in critical reviews and certain other non-
commercial uses permitted by copyright law.

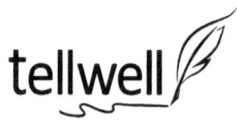

Tellwell Talent
www.tellwell.ca

ISBN
978-0-2288-2736-8 (Paperback)
978-0-2288-4066-4 (eBook)

Acknowledgments

Thank you to everyone who has played a pivotal role in the contribution of this book.

A special appreciation goes out to my Spouse for venturing into the unknown with me.

My Parents and Partners along the way.

Family (both sides), Friends, and Acquaintances.

My Progenies that inspire me to create a better World for them and others.

Thank you for your support, wisdom and willingness on all of our adventures we embarked on. Thanks to everyone who has shared an incredible space to listen and converse these ideas.

Table of Contents

The Pyramid 7
Introduction to the Cube 27
The Sphere of Operations 53
The Mirrored Universe 63
Conclusion 72
The What 79
Moving the Cube 82
Moving 84
Reflecting the Pyramid 97
Expanding the Sphere 103
The Allegory of the Two Best Friends. 112
Conclusion 117
The How 121
The Cube 125
The Pyramid 135
The Sphere 148
Conclusion 157

The Carousel

Someone dies (as any good story about the living goes), their soul meets Death and they cower for fear he has come to kill them. Death explains, "I can't kill you; you are already dead." The person asks, "Now what?" Death says, "It's your choice. What do you want to do?" The person thinks for a moment and says, "More time, I want more time." Death replies, "Time? You want more time? I'll give you more time," and like that Death snaps its bony fingers and turns the person into a developing fetus, and they go back into the cycle of birth, death, and rebirth with lifetimes ahead of them. They go through life fearing Death is waiting for them around every corner and behind every door, anticipating the inevitable. Death comes around again and again and the same meeting occurs, until one day, after a number of cycles long forgotten, Death asks again, "What would you like to do?" and the person replies, "I want to go with you."

– Geoff Hunnef

Introduction to the Three Centres

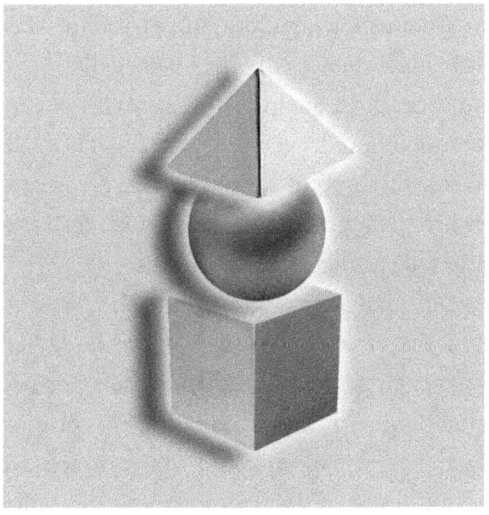

THIS BOOK IS ABOUT PERSONAL growth and development, and as such there are many different avenues we can invest ourselves into, but we are going to distill it all down to essentially three centres from which we engage reality: the body, the mind, and the heart. Pretty much everyone identifies with one of these areas, and in cultures all across the globe these three centres are acknowledged as being crucial for us to pay attention to for the overall health and quality of our lives. In traditional Chinese medicine and Tai chi, for example, they have what are called the "three treasures" located in the body: the lower *Dāntián*, or *Xià Dāntián*, is located roughly in the lower abdominal area and is connected to our physical health; the next going up is the middle, or the *Zhōng Dāntián*, located in the solar plexus and connected to our emotions and feelings; and the third is the upper, or *Shàng Dāntián*, located just above the brow line behind the forehead, connected to our thoughts and intellect. Anyone who had not cultivated their physical, mental, or emotional capabilities was seen as a poor individual, hence why they were called "treasures": if you had these three qualities you were considered to be a fortunate individual. It seems all aspects of life fall within one, two, or all three of these centres. No matter what we do in life through our thoughts, feelings, or actions, everything falls under these categories.

Conventionally, growing up in the West you are considered either artistic, athletic, or intelligent, and generally speaking, everyone thinks their perspective or way of engaging with the world is the best or most ideal, but in fact they are all equal, as you can achieve many great things in any of these three operating centres. But exceptional development in any one of these areas does not make for a fully developed human being. What do we mean by a "developed human being"? We are not just physical beings who exist in the Newtonian mechanics of the world, with no depth of connection to humanity or the intelligence to be able to see the value in intangible things. And just because you are able to compute the stars doesn't mean you can tie your shoes or feed yourself, and because you can relate to people doesn't mean you have the ability to help others. Development in all three areas is important and leads to a synergistic development that is greater than any one alone. Ultimately, it is in the development of these three areas that we start to be able to have more freedom in our lives, and begin to move with ever greater confidence in our competencies.

These three centres or operating systems are separate ways of engaging with existence. Each one has its own brain, so to speak, as we are not these things but the users of them. All tasks can be performed by any one of these brains, though it seems best to perform each task through the given centre.

Here's some examples to help illustrate what I mean:

The physical centre is best suited for physical tasks, and is not the same as muscle memory or a grooved pattern from repetition, such as the reloading of a rifle or the tying of one's shoes. It is a way of engaging with the world in a way that is different from using our minds. It becomes apparent to anyone who has ever been in a fight that thinking in thought is way too slow in the heat of battle. Things happen on a much more intuitive level—words and thoughts are too long and slow to activate. We have all experienced at some point or another finishing a paragraph without a clue as to what we just read. Or when we're trying to have a conversation with someone and maintain eye contact, offering verbal confirmation that we are in agreement with them, and by the end suddenly realizing we haven't the faintest idea of what they said. In both of these examples, we are trying to either comprehend something or relate to someone through the physical centre and achieving very little in the process.

The intellectual centre helps us navigate the world, using rational logic to help us foresee problems and find solutions through patterns and apply them skillfully. But when we use our minds to overthink a physical task, we get interrupted and trip over ourselves. We all know someone who is too up in their heads and not enough in their bodies when it comes to sex. Berman chemist Fritz Haber came up with a way to extract nitrogen from the atmosphere and enabled us to create fertilizer, providing food to countless people, but he also came up with and strategized the application techniques for mustard gas during World War I and was responsible for the loss of countless lives. Just because the mind has the ability to do something does not necessarily mean that thing should be done, and the ability to connect with humanity becomes ever more paramount as our intellectual capacities mount.

With the heart, the ability to connect and relate is crucial, not just for us on an individual basis, but a species as a whole. We will not move forward if we see ourselves as isolated and alone, as we can see the trauma that is inflicted upon people who are placed for long periods in solitary confinement. Take for example the horrifying Pit of Despair experiment by American psychologist Harry Harlow, where he would confine rhesus macaque monkeys into what was coined the "pit of despair." Shortly after birth, these monkeys were placed in solitary confinement in a cage for up to a year and starved of any contact with anyone, human or monkey, with devastating results. These monkeys are social creatures, and in the absence of the opportunity to socialize, they were traumatized. They would kill their young and were unable to socialize with other monkeys later in life, further perpetuating the isolation long after the bars and walls had been removed.

We are social creatures, and it seems in North America, there are metropolises where there are people surrounded by over a million other people who claim to have never felt lonelier. The bars and the walls aren't there, and yet we still have an inability to connect and relate to the people we live beside. If we don't learn to connect, perhaps much like the rhesus monkeys we may in the end turn on our young. But we all know we should not do business from an emotionally charged place, and we certainly don't want to receive a massage, dental work, or surgery from someone who just got off the phone after hearing some very heavy news.

The pursuit of personal growth, the intentional and applied development of all three centres, is our main goal with this book. Why we are talking about personal growth and development within these three centres, and why anyone would want to venture down this path in the first place, is simple: so that we can move through these three spaces of life—the intellectual, the physical, and the emotional worlds, with confidence in our competence.

To borrow an analogy from Armenian philosopher and spiritual teacher George Gurdjieff, the observer (the "I") sits inside a coachman-driven carriage being pulled by a team of horses. The observer who sits inside the carriage is largely unable to do much more than observe. The carriage represents the body, the physical form; the driver represents the mind, the intellectual form; and the horses represent the heart, the emotional form. The carriage, the driver, and the horse are all crucial components to the transportation of the passenger inside. The driver maintains the carriage, takes care of the horses, and directs and steers where the carriage goes to deliver the passenger. But the coachman is directionless without the passenger, unable to carry anyone without the coach, and won't be able to go anywhere without the horses. The carriage protects and carries the passenger and his luggage and supports the coachman while being led by the horses, and the horses, wild beasts that they are, can be powerful yet devastating if not handled properly. They can hurt people and damage property, and also themselves, so ideally, when moving through life, it is essential to have all these in check and developed so we can navigate with much greater ease and play.

The body spans the widest.

The mind sits the highest.

The heart lies the deepest.

For symbolic representation, we are going to break these centres into shapes, where the physical world is embodied in the cube, the mental sphere is crystalized in the pyramid, and the heart is represented in the sphere.

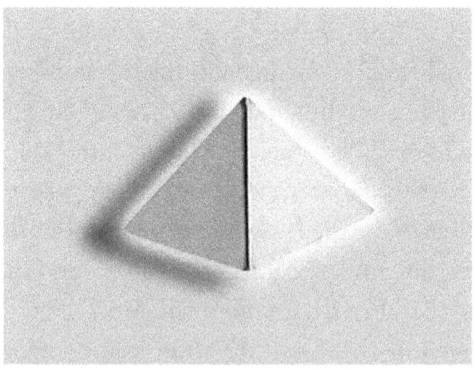

The Pyramid

Before moving forward, let's bear in mind it was once said by Aristotle, "It is the mark of an intelligent mind to entertain an idea without believing in it."

The world is full of ideas, and ideas are chairs we have never seen. When we close our eyes and imagine a chair, what does it look like? Does it have arms? Is it still a chair if there is no back? Is it on four legs, rockers, or wheels? Is it electric, does it kill? What about a bean bag chair? In this scenario, we see the idea of "chair" expand into a broad spectrum, from conventional structure and form to something that is literally a bag full of beans. In this little exercise, we see that as we get farther away from the original image, we get closer to a better understanding of the idea.

Reality is figuratively layers of chairs. The detailed information that we look into when looking at a chair depends on which one we are looking at. We can see that there are ideas within ideas. Stay with me—it's like the layering of visions. We could have an image of a dark alley at night. Across from the alley is a tree with a bush underneath. With regular vision, this is all we can see, while with night vision we may see a door at the end of the alley. With heat vision it is revealed there is someone behind the bush below the tree, while in broad daylight both of these layers may be rendered useless, making our regular vision best suited to the scene.

Each vision offers a glimpse of reality that the others were not privy to, and depending on the situation each one provides vital information to base your decisions and perceptions of reality on. The more layers of perspectives one can hold at any given time, the more options become available, and we are able to do more things with reality.

It's a good idea to collect many perspectives. It doesn't mean you have to believe in them, but you begin to be able to engage in the world in different ways. I asked my dad once if Spider-Man exists, to which he scoffed and replied with a matter-of-fact "of course not." I pointed out that we were both talking about a person, Peter Parker, who has a history and parents and aunts and uncles and an ongoing and evolving narrative. It is a movie franchise; kids want to be him; tons of money has been exchanged in his name. As much as Spider-Man does not exist, the idea certainly does, and just look at how much money can be made off someone who doesn't even exist. So keep in mind that things can exist in many different ways, and the way we perceive them can be many different things. The more layers you have, the more malleable reality becomes. The more rigid and singularly defined something is, the more locked in, rigid, and brittle reality becomes.

In the pursuit of collecting perspectives, we must layer over what is already standing. We must not delete, destroy, or remove and start anew, but add on and integrate with what has come before, changing it. As Sir Isaac Newton wrote in 1675, "If I have seen further it is by standing on the shoulders [sic] of giants." Far too often we are quick to throw the baby out with the bath water. When we disregard the old, it leaves us disconnected from our past, and the task of the new isn't to repeat the old.

Ideas are words, and a picture is worth a thousand words. A symbol has many pictures. A symbol that has continued to influence many great minds is the *Taiji*, which most people recognize and understand to be the symbolic representation of yin and yang, and to most lay people this symbol denotes dualism. But as we said, a picture is worth a thousand words, and there is much more being said than what is first perceived.

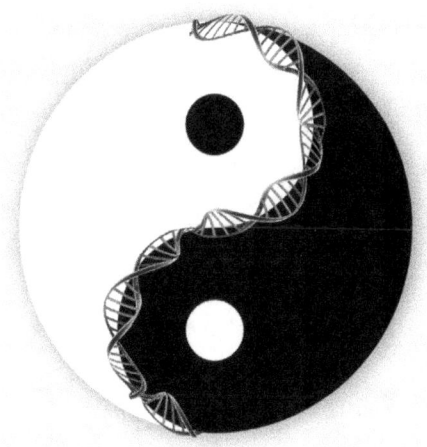

First let's begin with the most obvious. There is a distinct separation of two colours, often depicted as black and white. This is to represent the division in all things and ideas, past, present, and future, into two things. These two things are only ever in relation to other things; for example, if we were to define yin as cold and yang as hot and ask what 32 degrees Celsius is, hot or cold, it would be very difficult to say without it being defined by something else first, meaning 32 degrees Celsius is hot in relation to −2 degrees Celsius. But suddenly what was once hot becomes quite cool when the same 32 degrees Celsius is compared to the temperature required to boil water at sea level. Arguably, all things can be divided into two things when a comparison is made. For example with femininity and masculinity, as much as I am born a male a woman may be more masculine than I am, depending on what qualities, depending on what qualities we are comparing. But that doesn't make her a man, as she may be more feminine when compared to another woman. Here are a few cultural examples that could represent these ideas, all the while keeping in mind that everything could change at the drop of a hat.

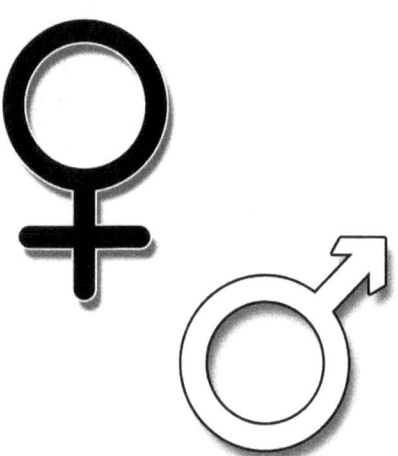

- yang-yin
- masculine-feminine
- weightlessness-heaviness
- thoughts-physical form

- up-down
- white-black
- right-left
- angles-curves
- direct-circuitous
- active-passive
- outside-inside

Secondly, consider the line that divides the two colours down the centre. The line is even, with equal amounts on either side, but not straight. This shows that at any given dissection of the image there may be more of one quality than the other, but there is an even amount of give and take on either side yielding a net zero in the total sum. This seemingly uneven balance is to convey that the harmony we are talking about is dynamic, not static, as nothing ever truly is. The line down the middle is curved as though a swirl is emanating from the centre, indicating movement, and the balance that occurs is due to the exchange between the two sides.

Let's take for example a bicycle wheel. One side is front and one side is back, or one side is yin and the other side is yang. When we stand the wheel upright and let go, it falls to one side, lifeless. But when there is a push and the exchange of front to back begins, and one becomes the other, movement occurs and balance appears. With either side of the wheel front and back, yin and yang, there is not one side that is better or more valuable than the other. They both play equal parts in making this moment happen. Think of a coin, with one side representing yin and the other side yang. Lying flat on either side, the coin is dead and motionless. But when we stand the coin on its edge and it stands in the space between either side, the coin can now spin and roll, dancing on both sides along the edge of yin and yang.

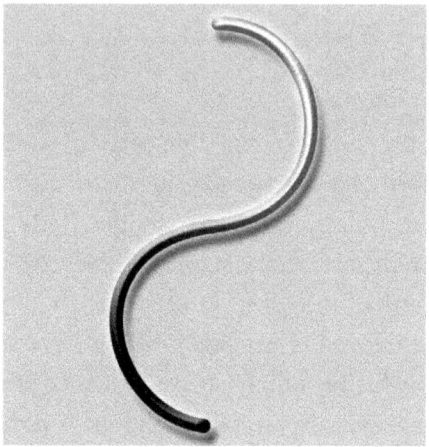

Third, we notice that the two divided colours are not squares, but curved and mirrored reflections of each other. As one grows the other shrinks in this mutual expansion and contraction, and in this we can see that as one grows larger and the other grows smaller, there comes a point where one side is at its most full and a sudden inversion occurs, and it becomes its opposite.

Not to get into views on morality, of right and wrong, but take for example the movie *Spotlight*, the 2015 American biographical drama which revealed the depth of knowledge and coverup that happened in the Roman Catholic Church regarding the abuse of children. The Catholic Church holds itself up as an exemplary model of morality and ethics, which certainly precludes the abuse of anyone, let alone children, and yet it harboured organizations within itself that promoted the very qualities that it denounced. Nietzsche once said, "Beware that, when fighting monsters, you yourself do not become a monster." It is possible to imagine a scenario where someone might justify the implementation of a curfew, routine checks, and invasion of privacy, all in the name of your safety.

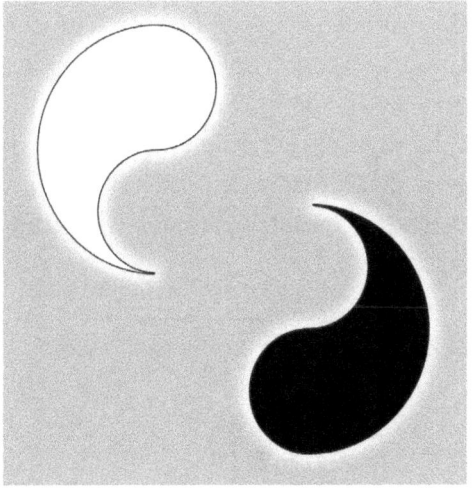

The fourth element in the Taiji symbol to touch on is the two dots of one colour found in the largest point of the other, showing that the seed of one is found within the belly of the other. I believe the saying "the poor will eat the rich" is a prime example how discontent leads to revolt, revolution, and change, all stemming from the oppression from the very people that instilled the discontent in the first place. From within itself it will produce its own antithesis. The very thing that is its opposite is often found within, as commonly we find that the thing we hate in others is the very thing we hate about ourselves.

Let us look at the story of the Buddha. Before Siddhārtha Gautama was born, his father heard that his son would not follow in his footsteps if he saw poverty, disease, and death. So when Siddhārtha was born, his father, a king, did everything in his power to keep his son inside the palace walls and shelter him from ever seeing these things. From the denial of the outside world, Siddhārtha pushed past his father's boundaries and ventured into the world, where he came upon poverty, disease, and death, and instead of becoming a ruler like his father he went on to become the Buddha, fulfilling the prophecy that his father tried so hard to prevent. The very thing that was meant to prevent is what produced the desire to discover.

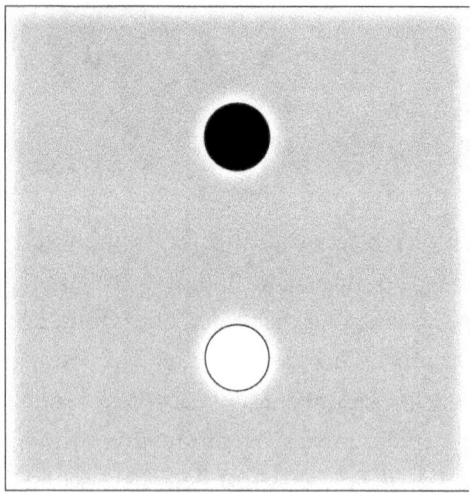

Perhaps the last thing to point out is that this image represents that two is actually only one. As much as there is yin and there is yang, they never exist alone as just yin and just yang. These two forces or ideas are more complementary than competitive, and they are much like a ball rolling: as one side rolls down the other side rolls up. Again, one side is no better than the other and it almost becomes impossible to exclude one direction from the other. Yet, in as much as those two directions are opposite, they work in complement due to the two existing as a whole. In short, all things are one thing and in that one thing are two things, but those two things make up the one.

Perhaps the best and most consistent representation of the idea of duality comes through the embodiment of sexuality and gender. In these concepts of femininity and masculinity, these ideas are often muddied by culture and frequently flip, change, and invert from culture to culture across the span of human history. For example, some cultures view the floor as masculine and the ceiling as feminine, and yet another culture perceives the inverse to be true. When we try to get to the heart of what lies across cultures and time as ubiquitously feminine and consistently masculine, this does not necessarily concern the depth of my voice, the broadness of my jaw, or the direction of my gaze.

In his book *A Brief History of Everything*, Ken Wilber highlights a definition that was put forth by a panel of anthropologists from around the world, which agreed cross-cultural masculinity identified itself through individualism and separateness, while femininity identified itself around the globe as communal and unified. In short, masculinity sees itself as being separate while femininity experiences itself as being together. Neither is wrong. Interestingly enough, this is the general stance most of us adopt: perceiving that we are all either connected and related or separate and disconnected, and of course the answer is probably both.

As we can see that the pursuit of balance is a desirable aim, it's evident that this objective is ever more difficult when we include the idea that balance is dynamic, alive, and ever-changing instead of static and dead. Life is full of paradoxes, and when we see how these things that seem to be at odds with each other actually work in tandem and together instead of against themselves, we begin to be able to do new and interesting things.

In the conscientious effort to move toward balance, here are five principles to observe when trying to cultivate a balanced development within all three of the centres or operating systems we use to engage with reality.

1. Finding your centre by defining your edge

In seeking balance, it is important to find the centre point of what you are balancing, but to do that you must first define the edges, the boundaries, and your end point. As William Blake wrote in *Proverbs of Hell*, "The road of excess leads to the palace of wisdom . . . You never know what is enough until you know what is more than enough." Rarely do we push our boundaries, but in making contact with and pushing into our edges, we see that the walls that were once in place start to move back, revealing a larger space for us to occupy, more of existence that we can engage with. Our world starts off small, but we can push the walls to grow to universal proportions.

To find one's edge we will look to an analogy called the Pitch-Black Room. Imagine you are brought to a pitch-black room where you have no bearings and no visual point of reference, and your task is to find the centre of the room. Without the aid of echolocation or night vision, how would we go about accomplishing this task? At the very least, we could start walking until we come to a wall. And then we could walk all the way to the other side. We could do this multiple times while counting out our footsteps until we had a pretty consistent measurement. In doing this, we will cross the midpoint multiple times to find the centre. Even after we have defined the length of the room, we may start to explore and define the width of the room, and to go even further, we could try to measure the height if we were so inclined. My point is, if we are to find the centre we will have to go to the edges, crossing our point of balance many times over before we find the sweet spot in the centre of the space we have mapped out. If the exit is in the centre of this room, we will only find it by stepping out of the five-foot radius that we are able to feel around us without moving. Until we are willing to step into the unknown, we never really know. Until we have gone to the end, we can't begin to define the centre. In finding the end points we start to have a better idea of the space we are trying to navigate.

When speaking of development, it is imperative to go beyond our comfort zone. As inspirational author John Assaraf once said, "A comfort zone is a beautiful place, but nothing ever grows there." In stepping into the unknown to explore and understand ourselves more, the greatest work comes from the places and the spaces we most dread venturing into. It is through exploring the difficult, the challenging, and the unpleasant that we begin to make the difficult easy, that we find the reward in the challenge and the comfort in the unpleasantness, and we begin to expand, now able to handle ever-greater hurdles that come our way. An African proverb says, "Smooth seas make for inexperienced sailors," and I think we are looking to sail the seas of life.

It is also vital to keep in mind that, to varying degrees, there are boundaries. We will encounter edges and end points, so it is useful to proceed with the overload principle: by using a slow, progressive, non-forced exposure to ever-greater intensity or complexity, we grow in our thoughts, in our bodies, and in our hearts. We rarely push ourselves to our limit, usually living instead in a prison built of our fears of the unknown. To know one's self best is to seek choppy water. To develop the mind, you don't have to take up music lessons or learn complex mathematics, though they are phenomenal practices to train and develop the mind—the mind in the context of the paradigms and perspectives of reality.

One way to do this is to seek out and attempt to understand new and different perceptions of reality. Expose yourself to things you don't understand by applying the great inversion principle, first written about by Carl Gustav Jacob Jacobi, a German mathematician who has contributed greatly to the development and understanding of elliptic functions, differential equations, dynamics, determinants, and number theory. When asked how he was able to find solutions to some of the greater problems, he proclaimed, "Invert, always invert." He would recommend writing the equation backwards, and in doing so new things would arise that lend themselves to new solutions previously unseen. In the pitch-black-room analogy, the inversion principle in play would be in walking to the opposite side of the room, and having done that, beginning to gain a new understanding of what you are trying to perceive. When you flip upside down, things suddenly become very confusing, but if you don't panic and let things settle and your mind's eye adjust, you start to see things you didn't quite see before. The next step is to integrate the two polarities, as we do not exist at either end of extremes but rather the space between the two.

Ideas arise from matter, like watching a log roll down a hill. This may give rise to the idea of a wheel. When we also cast our ideas onto matter, we can give certain inanimate objects special properties, like a childhood stuffed bear, or we can project past traumas onto unassociated people we currently know, and in this way we begin to notice that our environment and experiences shape us both inside and out. With that it becomes extremely interesting to explore the thought that we can shape our environment, and in turn we can shape and change ourselves. As we push our boundaries our understanding of our shape changes, and as our shape changes our centre shifts. This is how we change ourselves both inside and out. It seems we are so vast in the depths of ourselves that we may never come to fully understand who we are, as we seem to keep going ever farther beyond what we thought was possible, and what we thought could be real.

2. Tension and relaxation

To produce movement one must create tension; to create tension one must first relax. To relax, one must first be tense.

Tension and relaxation in the mind are very useful, but both seem to be at odds with the other, keeping in mind that things are much more in between the poles of the situation, rather than at one end or the other. In regard to the mind and its comprehension of reality, there have been analogies using the term "grip," as in, "I need to get a grip on reality," or "I'm losing my grip on reality." Rock climbers encounter a similar experience in their field, and they use the term "optimal grip" to describe the nuance between too much and too little. If you hold on too tight you get stuck and can't move onward and upward, and if your grip is too loose, you're likely to lose your holding as well as yourself. To continue further with this analogy, the only way to climb up is to let go then grab on, and repeat this all the way. We fight to let go and we fight to hold on. When we learn to navigate this space, it becomes easier to know when to hold on and when to let go. When our understanding of reality is too tense, too fixed, too rigid, too set with how we think, we become susceptible to crumbling from the tension that keeps us fixed and brittle when we encounter the ever-changing and dynamic rollercoaster that existence is. As strong as the mighty oak may be, it is the willow that weathers the storm.

Tension in the mind allows us to focus, but too much tension and we get tunnel vision and lose sight of the whole. Remain in a lax daydream state and we miss the tiger in the bushes. Where is the exchange and interplay between laser focus and ingeniously creative meanderings?

Neither one is better, and much like the ball they work in favour of the other. To remain only in one state will be our downfall.

A number of years ago, there was an experiment on a Daily Planet episode where they were tracking eye movements looking at a striking image between people who were born and raised in the Far East compared to people who were born in the Far West. What they found when presented with a picture of a tiger leaping out of the forest at the onlooker was that the Westerners' eyes mainly fell upon the tiger, the seemingly obvious threat, and a little around the peripheral, while when people from the East looked at the same picture their eyes mainly fell upon the peripheral. When asked why the test subjects were looking where they were, the general response was that the tiger was obvious; they were more interested in the exits or options around. Interestingly, when you put the centre and the peripheral together you end up with a whole picture. When we are able to hold both the concepts of tension and relaxation in mind at the same time, new and interesting things become apparent.

3. Change and the same

When we read a new book or reread an old one, two different things happen. When we reread an old book we become more familiar with the characters, the story becomes more engrained, and we even start to see new things or discover deeper or hidden meanings, while when we pick up a new book there are new characters, a different plot, and unseen twists. A whole new world opens up to be discovered, and this is not to say either one is better. I am reminded of an essay written by William Ralph Inge titled "Some Wise Saws," which contains the adage: "There are two kinds of fools. One says, "This is old, therefore it is good"; the other says, "This is new, therefore it is better." Both have use and both can be a hinderance, but we need both. We need consistency and reliability in our world, constants to help us orient, align, and familiarize, but we are also in a constantly changing world that is rarely ever the same.

The value of being consistent is that it allows us to commit to a process. It's what gets a daunting task done; it's how every great thing that was ever undertaken came to completion. Consistency of character helps you to be a reliable individual, as there are many people who will flip-flop with commitments, saying yes one minute and then back out the next, making deciding on plans frustrating. You can build trust with consistency and you can do a lot with trust. But consistency can also make you predictable, like the example of the re-watched movies or reread books, when the plot becomes foreseeable and there are no more surprises. Similarly in chess, when the outcome of the game can be seen and a checkmate is called, even though it may be three or four moves down the line. Both players choose not to play through to the end and opt to start a new game. It is the uncertainty in any good experience that keeps us drawn in, and yet in our lives we strive so hard to produce a certainty, which brings us more to a point of stagnation than a place of safety. Our safety becomes a prison which eventually becomes a tomb.

Doing things the same way allows for a deep study and understanding of the thing you are invested in, but anything done too long becomes detrimental, just like eating the same food over time will cause the flavour to fade, and what was once a delight will now fill you with disgust. Consistency allows you to build and create success, but it is diversity that is the spice of life. Variety provides different experiences; as we begin to experience different things we perceive new ideas, and it can add layers of perspective instead of presenting only the one story. By reading many stories instead of one, you may start to see the idea of archetypes instead of a simple character, or the shapes of stories instead of the plot development of only one. Even when trying to convey a concept to someone, sometimes one analogy doesn't work, but someone else walking by could casually make a comment and suddenly the recipient grasps the idea that you just couldn't get across. It shows that approaching things from different angles can offer greater progress than consistently ramming at the same spot.

There is value in consistency and it is important to bring in variation, so I am suggesting that things exist in the space between rather than either one alone, and so we are trying to find the balance between doing the same thing differently and doing different things the same.

4. Make a pattern, break a pattern

Patterns are all around us, from the set pattern in your scheduled routine to the circadian or menstrual cycles in our bodies, to the seasons of the year, or to astrological events like eclipses. Patterns allow us to predict the world around us, to establish routines in our days to bring order and stability to our lives. As the Israeli athlete Israeli athlete and trainer Ido Portal has said, "The tools we use to build us become the very tools we use to destroy us." Unfortunately, the patterns that can help us get established and ahead in life when practiced to an extreme can become our very downfall. We get too caught up in the idea that this one thing is everything. The more we repeat something, the more we get locked into it, and we see fewer and fewer options. And patterns are not all good either, as we can have patterns set in our behaviours that are undesirable. Whether it's an addiction to a substance or an experience, or repetitive negative self-talk, there can be all sorts of negative patterns that we don't care to carry with us.

The making of patterns can help accomplish great things, but it can also become the source of our despair. It is important to remember we are not these patterns, but rather what exists outside of them, and this is why it is important to not only make patterns but to also regularly break them. It can be very helpful to see beyond the patterns that we can become so fixated on.

When we first look at the world, it seems to be a mess, a chaotic swirl of everything, but then in the madness of this maelstrom patterns begin to arise and help to secure this insanity into some kind of predictable outcome, allowing us to feel safer, thinking we know what is coming next. The problem comes when we get too attached to any of these patterns. We begin to think, *Hey, if it's gotten me this far, it will continue to get me further.* Except it doesn't. What worked for us at one time may not work at another.

If we are existing in a world of chaos and confusion, exposing ourselves to order and routine would do us a world of good. If we live in an existence of high routine and order, we tend to come more alive when we step out into the great unknown.

5. Work and play

Play is to exploring as work is to building. It is incredibly valuable to work on building yourself, your perspectives, your body, your mind, and your relationships. It is also important to play: with our minds, our bodies, and our hearts. As we do, we begin to play with the perspectives of our lives, and we begin to play with the possibilities of who we can become.

The diligent and consistent application of focused work can yield great things. Just ask any chess champion or gold-medal Olympian and they will tell you that their focused and applied efforts contributed greatly to the acquisition of their highly developed skills, yet often at a significant cost.

Work pays the bills. It is often associated with productivity and success, while play has been seen as something to be relegated to childhood and left behind. As we stepped into adulthood it was time to put away such childish endeavors, but there are things within play that are as valuable as work. There is more power in approaching a negotiation with a playful attitude than with the use of stern logic alone.

There is value in work and there is discovery in play—how do we straddle both? How do we find play within work and work within play?

When we are able to approach the seriousness of work with a playful attitude, we are more relaxed with the task and are more likely to see things that may otherwise be missed with a fixed gaze. We can see that something as frivolous and self-indulgent as play embodies things as valuable as work. As previously mentioned, we are not *things* but *between* things, and to stay in one you lose the other, so be like the coin and dance along the edge.

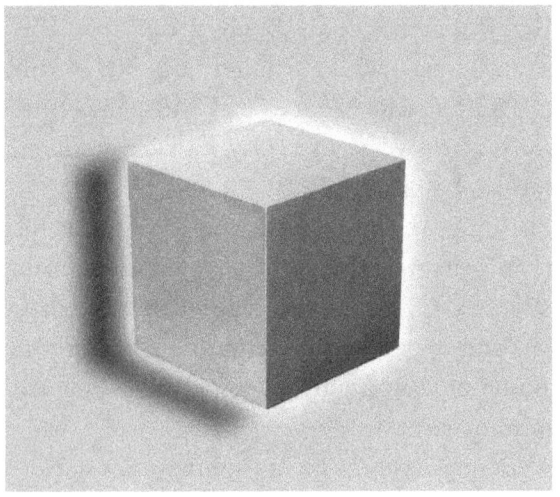

Introduction to the Cube

ONE OF THE MOST OBVIOUS ways we engage with the world is in the physical sense of things. We all have a body and we all use it to physically navigate space. Movement is a crucial aspect of our lives; research shows the benefits exercise has on the body through improved coordination, increased strength, prolonged stamina, better body composition, greater self-confidence, and elevated mood. It also helps with depression, heart disease and many other physical ailments.

Movement is crucial to our health beyond just how we appear in the mirror or perform on the field. For instance, the lymphatic system is essentially our tissues' drainage mechanism, aiding in the removal of cellular waste, but unlike the cardiovascular system—where the heart pumps blood through our arteries, capillaries and veins even when we are lying there doing nothing—the lymphatic system requires the aid of mechanical action. The lymphatic system relies on us to move our bodies around, compressing and stretching and moving in deep ranges to squeeze the tissue to compress them and help move the fluids between chambers.

Reality is super strange, and to illustrate the depth that our bodies demand movement to be healthy, we will consider our skin. Our skin is an organ; it is alive and responds to its environment. If we were to remain immobile for long periods, our bodies will actually open up and start to merge with their surroundings. *Ridiculous*, I hear you say, *that sounds crazy!* It's true. When a patient is in a coma, nurses will routinely come in and move them around because of bedsores, which occur when your body starts to open up and attach itself to the material that it is next to, absorbing it into itself, and if someone in a coma doesn't move, their skin will begin to merge with the bedsheets, and then you have a real mess. A real-life example was in an NBC News article dated 3/12/2008 in Kansas, about a woman who sat on her boyfriend's toilet for two years. When help was finally called in, the woman had to be transported to the hospital along with the toilet seat, which had become fused to her. My point is that movement is deeply connected to our experience of existence, whether it is of the mind, the body, or the heart. Movement is part and parcel of existence, experience, and life, and it is with our bodies that we physically connect to the idea of movement.

Now, keep in mind the idea of collecting perspectives, or lenses, that we spoke about earlier in this book. The way we perceive our bodies influences the way we move. When I ask people to describe how they visualize their bodies, they tend to describe something like a stick figure. In that image you are trying to move something that you perceive as a two-dimensional object that is actually a three-dimensional object moving in a four-dimensional space, and in that we quickly lose something which produces a movement that is more akin to a clunky flip-flop than the roll of a ball. As much as we may think we have an understanding of our form, the image and idea of our body has taken many variations and is still in a current revision of understanding even now. We look at the body through the lens of culture, and even in these modern times we are still discovering and understanding new things about the body all the time. When collecting and overlapping perspectives of the body, we can see what mankind was looking at and what we thought was important from artwork and depictions in anatomy charts from our past. As we pass through cultures across time and space on this planet, we can see the hyper-detail of the musculature, as in the anatomical works of Juan Valverde de Amusco (circa 1560 C.E.) You can see that it is through the function of our muscles that we shift our eyes, turn our heads, and extend our arms. These are the things that help us interact and engage with the world around us.

When we move to the Middle East during the 1400s we can see in the imagery contributed by Mansūr Ibn Ilyās from Persia the heavy attention given to the vascular and digestive systems, where the thought was something to the effect of "cool, great, muscles do all those wonderful things, but you could lose an arm and still be fine." If the blood stops flowing or you puncture a lung or the digestive system backs up, major systemic failure ensues and things go south fast.

When we go to India as far back as 1500–500 BCE, we find writings in texts called the *Rigveda* describing *chakras*. These energetic centres influence and control a variety of functions that range from the physical to the emotional and spiritual. When we move farther east to

China, we encounter the meridian systems, which describe and depict flows of energy through channels that are shown in drawings dating as far back as the 1500s, while in Taoism they show the entire universe inside the body. And if we head to South America, where the indigenous tribal shamans speak of the body with an aura extending out from it (which looks like a bristly egg), we can bring this right up to modern times, where Thomas Myers has been able to show in his book *Anatomy Trains* that the fascial system has structures in it that were previously undiscovered, with striking similarities to the meridian systems in the East. There has also been a change in the way we envision the heart as recently as 2011, from four chambers attached together to one sheet that wraps around itself, producing what is called the "helical heart," shaped like a spiral, supposedly creating more of a pull in the system than a push. Discoveries like this may influence the way we make pacemakers or even pumps.

I am not saying any of these are better or worse than the others, I am merely pointing to the idea that there are many ideas to the form of our body, and the way we perceive ourselves influences the way we move and interact with our bodies. The more layers we are able to hold at any given moment, the more options or ways of engaging with our physical world we have.

As much as I postulated that we have never seen a chair, I would put forward the idea that we have never seen our body. We have seen from across cultures and time many ideas of the body, from being the muscle just under the skin to the depth of organs and bones, to systems and things that can't physically be seen or found in the body, like the chakras and meridian channels to the universe inside to energetic bristles extending outside the body. There have been many understandings and perceptions of the body to be aware of, and as we include the layers new things become available.

When looking at the development of the physical body, there are some concepts that can be useful to include while pursuing development in this centre.

1. The centre and edge of our physical existence

We literally exist between the physical space that is our centre and the edge of what we define as self. Frequently we encounter things within ourselves that feel set, stuck, immovable, or immutable, and, surprisingly, more often than not all sorts of things within the body can and do change. The fact is that when you bring your intentions and efforts toward things, those things that once seemed so set begin to morph and change.

For example, within the application of physical development for sports there is what is known as the "overload principle," whereby constantly exposing ourselves to difficult or challenging things sees our body adapt and change to the stimuli that it is exposed to. By lifting heavy weights, we begin to be able to lift heavier weights. By performing complex patterns, we begin to grasp and replicate those patterns. By running fast, we begin to run faster. We can shape bones and muscles, our nervous system, and our sensitivity by exposure to ever-greater intensities and complexities of situations, and it is through this we become more capable and savvy enough to be able to navigate through the physical world.

Our bodies become better at doing anything that they do or don't do. It's not just a matter of "if you don't use it you lose it," it's, "the more we do, the more we can do, while the less we do, the less we can do." The more that we move, the more that we can move; inversely, the less that we move the less that we can move. The more we move, the more our bodies make moving more efficient and easier, and the more we sit the more our bodies make sitting easier.

Let's get back to the proverbial pitch-black room. If we only ever stay to one side of the room, never venturing beyond what is known, the space that we move in or exist in is only half of what it could be, while the more of the room we explore, the more of the room we have confidence and competence to move in, our world becomes bigger, and we are able to do more things. This is why it is so important to explore our boundaries to find out what we are really working with. We see with physical development what is a wall today might be removed tomorrow, because as we encounter our barriers, we begin to find the strength to push past them.

But this approach is taken through slow and progressive exposure, as we don't achieve the ability to squat 225 kg from day one. We slowly load, allowing the body and the mind to adapt to what it is being exposed to. If we take a typical untrained sixteen-year-old and put him under that weight, there is a very good chance the kid is not making his way up from the descent of that squat without a high chance of injury. What can harm you today could make you stronger tomorrow, but as with all things, context is extremely important. There is a man named Steve Ludwin in the States who is not only a snake handler, bitten a large number of times by venomous snakes, but he has gone so far as to regularly inject himself with a concoction of snake venom, and by this has seemingly built up a tolerance to a number of snake venoms. His blood is now being used by researchers from the University of Copenhagen, where Dr. Brian Lohse, an associate professor in chemical and molecular biology, is looking into using Ludwin's blood to find the antibodies that could be used in future antivenom serums. This is to illustrate that something at high doses would seem likely to cause harm but when a low and slow exposure happens over time, the body is more than capable of handling it. Our bodies have a phenomenal capacity to adapt and we can consciously use that to our advantage, where instead of waiting for an issue to come along and then hope the body is able to adapt and change to the demands, we pre-emptively develop ourselves so that we are better able to deal with the challenges that lie ahead.

We can make our bones harder; our muscles bigger and stronger; our movements faster, more precise, more complex, and simpler. There are many ways to develop our physical sense, and at the very heart of existence it seems the physical world is the most fundamental element. As rudimentary as that may seem, it is the basics that win the game. It's the foundation that everything else sits upon. If you build on shaky ground, don't expect to have a structure that lasts for too long. Our physical body is a fundamental keystone to our existence. Simply put, if it stops working, everything that sits on top of it collapses. If the body begins to fail, everything else will fail. In the horse, carriage, and driver analogy, if the carriage breaks down the horses can't pull it, and the driver can't direct the horses to bring the carriage to the passenger's desired destination. The physical body holds and supports the other two spheres the heart and the mind, if the body fails our emotions and our mind will soon follow.

Our physical health plays a huge role, as we know that an active body tends to be a healthy body, and less likely to be affected by—but not immune to—diseases like diabetes and heart disease to name a few. It certainly goes a long way toward staving off obesity, but it also plays a crucial role in our mental health, as a healthy body tends to lend itself toward a healthier mind. When it comes to matters of the heart, it can play a tremendous part in the relationship with ourselves and the confidence we exude from being in our skin. As much as we are not about body shaming, I have heard from many people that, after some time within their relationships, their partners stopped caring for themselves in the same way they once did, and they became less physically attracted to them. This can certainly put an added strain on a relationship, and so it seems that by using, stretching, and challenging the body in all sorts of ways, we are able to keep it more vibrant, youthful, and healthy.

In 1991, in Oracle Arizona, Biosphere 2 was constructed, a miniature closed ecosystem that was meant to mimic the earth's environment. One thing came as a surprise. As the foliage continued to develop inside the biosphere, the scientists were noticing they were having a hard time with the trees, as they were having difficulty staying up and would keep falling over. After investigating this further, it was unearthed that in the construction of the biosphere one of the few factors that hadn't been taken into account was wind. On Earth, the constant movement of the wind on foliage was enough of an environmental cue to stiffen up and reinforce the fibres of the trees, allowing them to grow to the heights that they do.

We cannot live on the edge, nor can we stay were we started, but there seems to be a dance in the space between the two we can participate in as we venture outward and return to recover. A common saying in the training world is, "You don't grow in the gym, you grow in your sleep," but if you don't expose yourself to the stimuli during the day your body will not grow when it sleeps at night. In the context of relationships, we push our boundaries ever farther outward into uncharted territory and head home to familiarity and comfort. If we stay in either one for too long, bad things happen, but when we venture back and forth we allow for growth and move the span of our capabilities to ever-deeper heights.

2. Tension and relaxation of the physical body

Within the body, one of the main features or abilities we have access to from a very early point in our existence is movement. Our bodies are what allow us to literally move through the physical world. It is perhaps one of the most rudimentary ways we interact with the world, and yet it is certainly one of the most profound ways we can express ourselves. We use our bodies to move through our daily activities, such as fuelling ourselves through eating, not to mention procuring the food to do so, but even our breath and the circulation of our cardiovascular system to the lymphatic system requires movement. We fight, we fuck, we build, we live through movement.

Tension manifests in neurologically innervated, activated, and excited tissue. Muscles work via the brain, sending a signal down the spinal column through the nervous system to a motor unit, which consists of a single motor neuron and all the muscle fibres it innervates and activates. The size of the unit can involve only a few muscle fibres—for fine movements like writing, suturing, or eye twitching—to very large numbers of muscle fibres, for activities like walking, weightlifting, or wrestling. In some of the more profound examples of tension at either end of the spectrum, we find *hypotonicity*, where the muscle recruitment is weak. Few fibres are recruited, and moving around feels lethargic and cumbersome due to the sheer amount of willpower it takes to get around. Hypertonicity constantly activates a high number of muscle fibres, and they too find moving strenuous and difficult but for the opposite reason: there is too much tension not letting go. When the muscle fibres stay recruited, they push against the closing of the joints, against their movement, making it difficult to move, as they are often fighting with themselves to get into position.

Our ability to produce tension is extremely important, but just as important is the ability to let it go. The very tension that we use to be able to move, to manipulate, and to articulate ourselves through life can also become a prison, locking us ever more into ourselves . . . literally. The more tension we carry in our body, the stiffer, more rigid, immovable, and brittle become. When there is too little tension causes us to become ineffective in the world.

Tension in the body does not form merely as a product of our attempts to move our bodies; it can arise from overuse, underuse, and disease, as well as physical, mental, and emotional stressors and traumas.

What happens in our bodies also happens in our minds, and what happens in our minds happens in our bodies. We can observe the body-mind connection quite easily. When pain arises in the body, it registers in the brain. Under MRI and CT scans we can see what is called a typical pain response, where if I am poked with a needle in my foot we can see it register in the scan of the brain. To illustrate how we can see it in the reverse, where tension starts in the brain and manifests in the body, imagine a situation where a person in a stressful situation, like negotiating a contract or experiencing a moment of frustration. It is common to see the shoulders tense and rise into a shrug. When someone else walks by, notices the raised shoulders, gives the traps a squeeze, and says "relax," the tense person's mind is brought both to the awareness of tension and the physical location of its manifestation. With awareness, the tense person may be able to instantly drop the mounting tension by bringing their mind to it and consciously letting it go.

There are varying degrees of tension and our awareness of it, from acute and very immediate tension, like an injury or a muscle spasm, where you become hyper-aware of the contraction, to much more subtle micro-contractions and holding patterns that most people are unaware of until someone pokes them where the tension resides, much like a trigger point. Without this alert, the tension that has slowly built can be there for a long time and become chronic.

The progression of tension in the body starts off very subtly. Someone may notice the tension if the tissue where the tension is located is pressed on. If nothing is done, tension accumulates and the person may only begin to notice discomfort when stressing the tense area, through exercising or strenuous activity. If nothing is done, the tension starts to show up in regular daily activity, such as putting on a coat, doing up a seat belt, or pulling up pants. If it is still not dealt with, the pain from the tension starts to affect the person's sleep, where they might wake up in the night due to pain in the area of tension, and if left unchecked the pain eventually becomes evident in your consciousness, day or night.

Similar to the analogy above of the person becoming stressed at work and then consciously letting it go after having their awareness cued. Just the same, it's evident in the physical body where tension in the body can manifest in the mind. One way to address the existing tension in your body is by becoming aware of it—if you don't know that there is a problem, why would you try to fix it? Constantly contracted tissue in your body not only weakens you by making the muscles unavailable, but it also restricts and weighs you down, making the subjective experience of moving your body heavier.

Good healthy tissue is unresponsive tissue. When someone pokes you and there is an uncontrolled response where you move, grimace, moan, or feel ticklish, these are all signs of tension in the tissue. Healthy tissue is unresponsive and intelligent. It doesn't just lie there anticipating a broken bone, and it doesn't move you to laughter or discomfort from a simple poke or prod.

We don't grow in the gym, but in our sleep, when we are relaxed. This is when we physically change, unless there was no stress from the tensions that we encounter in our day. Again, it isn't one or the other but the exchange between the two that develops ourselves.

3. Between consistency and variability with the physical body

WHEN DEVELOPING OUR PHYSICAL FORM, whether it be in the pursuit of aesthetics or performance, it has been observed through exposure to a stimulus that doing something once doesn't necessarily provide adequate information, environmental cues, and experience to induce significant physical changes, including neurological adaptations. We require repeated exposure to grasp the idea or to give the body the proper cues to adapt in decisive ways. That is to say, if the goal is to increase the weight we use while doing squats, performing them once every six months is probably not enough of an environmental cue to drive the body to adapt in such a way as to accommodate the new and frequent demands. It is costly to add on to the body or to make improvements, and so if the body doesn't have to keep something it will get rid of it. If you don't use it, you lose it. Too much energy goes into the maintenance of muscle when there is no need for it. This is why an attractive body is often a healthy body, and a healthy body is one that is being used regularly, one that is in demand and being challenged and growing to the capabilities of overcoming those challenges. I am not talking about attractiveness in regard to muscularity or leanness, but people who move well tend to look good. We also understand that what looks "good" is subjective, but health has never really been out of vogue, and through all the years of what may or may not be considered attractive, movement has been beautiful and a body that moves well tends to look attractive. So staying dedicated to a regular and frequent movement practice is crucial, as we use our bodies all the time. It is something of ours that is being used every day, and it could use regular attention to an explorative and developmental practice.

When we do something over and over again, we begin to naturally refine the action or task. We become more efficient with our movements. Let's take running as an example. If we took up running, the amount of calories that are used to run the distance of one kilometre over the span of a year will decrease at the end of that year, even without an attempt to improve our gait or consciously focusing on improving any aspect of the movement. Just run for a year and you will naturally improve the efficiency of your run.

We can see why repetition and staying committed to something allows us to accomplish great things, just as building great structures to withstand the tests of time requires an investment of time and a commitment to stay on task until completion. As with the physical form, the classic example of this would be men in North America and the bench press: a big chest and a high weight load to go with that chest is a hot pursuit for many. Of course, we would start with the bench press (a classic decision), and, knowing that if you want to build something great you have to stay committed and consistent, we stay committed to the bench press by consistently hitting it three times a week. Three years later, our pectorals "pecs" are looking bigger, our bench weight is significantly higher, people are complimenting us on the weight of the bar—things are going great. Except lately our shoulder and right arm have started to present a constant ache, and it hurts to put a seat belt on or to pull up our pants, and at night we can barely sleep because the pain keeps us up. Our shoulders have slouched and our posture has caved in and it really hurts to bench press and the doctor says to stop benching. And suddenly we can't hear anything else the doctor has to say. We can't stop bench pressing—look at all the success we have gained from it: the respect in the gym, the looks from the girls or guys, the comments from friends, a sense of pride and confidence in our physical capabilities . . . it has gotten us all this. And we'll lose it all if we stop. So we continue to bench, locked into a destiny with a sinking ship. Recalling again Ido Portal's maxim about the tools we use to build: when all we have is a hammer, it is surprising how much everything starts to look like a nail.

So, if repetition builds, which is desirable but has inherent flaws from the very thing that it builds, how do we build while avoiding the same pitfalls? It seems variation offers itself as a remedy for ailments that arise from consistency.

There are injuries that occur consistently within certain sports. Long-distance runners will generally share a more common type of injury due to the repeated movements. Cyclists will typically have issues with their hips, knees, and neck. Easy examples would be golfers and tennis players. Golfers will typically get golfer's elbow, which is often experienced as pain on or around the medial epicondyle or the inside of the elbow, while tennis players, because of the backhand swing, tend to develop tennis elbow, which is found on the other side along the lateral epicondyle, or outside of the elbow. Both create pain in the elbow, but golfers will rarely develop something akin to tennis elbow, largely because they don't use a backswing. Coaches have learned to cross train in the offseason, having their athletes do activities either completely different from their sport or different but the same, as in utilizing a different environment but performing the same activity. For example, if we were to take a professional snowboarder and have them spend three months skateboarding and then three months surfing, the actions are similar—balancing on a board in motion—but by changing the environment there are a whole bunch of novel lessons that are picked up and applied more generally to a different context.

It has been said that if you want to be good at something you should have many teachers. If you want to be a good fighter, spar with lots of different fighters; if you want to be a good dancer, dance with lots of different partners. Every teacher provides a personal angle on a particular subject, and, as we have discussed earlier, if you are able to pick up layers of lenses from each person you begin to have more tools in the toolbox, and you begin to see more options, more possibilities. When variability is brought into training, it can help break past previous plateaus; heal injuries brought on from repetitive strain; help to redistribute muscular tension across joints; and bring excitement, intrigue, and focus back into training. Good coaches encourage their athletes to cross train in the offseason. They recommend doing something that breaks out of the set patterns that their sport applies, but it is not recommended to take a season off.

There is a paradox presented by the longevity of practice: the more you do something and the longer you do it, the more difficult it can become to maintain, whether it's from injury, time constraints, or even sheer boredom of the practice. Doing anything for long periods can become difficult. So how do we do the same thing over and over while managing the stressors and boredom that can ensue?

We should look to the elite high-level performers, as they are the ones who are putting themselves through the highest levels of exposure to long periods of intense training. Outside of genetics, most of the top competitors are relatively cool, calm, and relaxed people. They know how to manage their stress, as this can derail training with injuries and sickness. But they were also doing something extremely creative in their pursuits. They have figured out how to do the same thing in as many different ways as possible, and as they explore variations they discover new weaknesses or insights that help set them apart from their contemporaries.

We often get caught up in things rather than ideas. Physically, when we repeat anything over time it becomes problematic. At one point that thing was useful but perhaps it no longer is, yet we hold on, thinking that it has gotten us to a certain point and it will take us to the next. As we begin to be exposed to the many different ways that people move, we begin to build our own kinetic matrix of how movement occurs, and to see that we are not these things but rather the spaces between these things.

4. The making and breaking of patterns

Our lives embody patterns from major celestial events like the solar and lunar eclipses, as well as global patterns, from the passing of seasons, menstrual cycles, and circadian rhythms to the patterns of our interactions with other people and our own thoughts. Patterns have the potential to free us and they have the power to enslave us. It is up to us where we fall on that line.

When it comes to physical development, establishing patterns—which could also be read as "habits"—can often be that which makes or breaks us, from the patterns of our morning routines to the types of food, its quantity, and the times we eat to our training routines and rehearsals, or the lack thereof. It is important to remember that patterns are perspectives and perspectives are ideas and ideas are tools, and we are looking to increase our toolbox. We are not these patterns but the space between these patterns.

From a physical level regarding the development of the body, doing something once doesn't really give the body enough stimuli to make adequate changes, and so a repetition begins. As soon as you do something more than once, a pattern starts to form. It can be extremely useful to bring order and patterns into our lives, from making our beds in the morning to having a regular sleep schedule and movement practice. We can see many of these patterns instilled in military training. The military is a place people can go if they want to develop more structure and discipline in their lives, as these are the foundations of many of the greats. Even patterns of movement that have been rehearsed can free the mind to focus on other things while the body performs a well-rehearsed movement. Much like learning to walk as a child, or a patient learning to walk again after coming out of a coma, it can take an exhausting amount of energy to think our way through each step. By the time we are thirty-four years old, we have mastered this skill to such a degree that we can be walking while talking on the phone and chewing gum while trying to figure out what to order for lunch. It can become so automatic that it can afford us new spaces to bring thought and awareness into.

Patterns can also cause issues, as we already covered that repeating anything for long periods tends to produce undesirable effects. These undesirable patterns could be as simple as inefficient holding patterns of our form, whether we are running or fighting. A common beginner's posture tends to be a sort of *kyphotic* crunch, or a rounding of the back, hunching forward in posture, while more experienced athletes take on a more upright and aligned position where the spine is straighter, allowing for a more efficient and less inhibited flow of the neurological impulse to flow from the spine out to the motor unit along the central nervous system. It can manifest in the gait of your run, if there is a dropped hip or a collapsed knee and contribute to patterns that produce an inefficiency to even larger aspects. As with martial arts, each of the styles has a pattern that can lock you into a predictability that can lead to the loss of a fight.

There are all sorts of styles within martial arts and fighting, from Boxing, Brazilian jiu-jitsu, Karate, Kenpō, Sambo, Kung fu, Silat, Systema, Krav Maga, Muay Thai . . . and the list goes on. Within all of these, each participant will adopt a particular posture, stance, or form, and there are patterns and ideas in all of them. They are all perspectives and ideas of movement in regard to interaction with another human being in a combative relationship. All offer different tools. We collect perspectives as we seek to learn a form, adhere to it, practice it in its pure form . . . and then kill it. Break the pattern and change it to something else. As we go along, we are looking to become formless, something unrecognizable, something unpredictable. Much like chess, if your opponent in a combative experience can start to see what you are doing they can start to anticipate and predict your next move. They can set you up toward failure as they become more aware of your next step.

The more we do something, the more we take on the identity of or alignment to that one thing. Bodybuilding is great; they have figured out fantastic protocols for hypertrophy, which is the enlargement of an organ or tissue (in this case muscle tissue) in size of its cells, and their understanding of nutrition and supplementation were far ahead of the times. Powerlifters have mastered ridiculous feats of strength in the bench press, squat, and deadlift, while weightlifters have been able to throw tremendous weights from the ground up overhead in the blink of an eye. CrossFit's intensity is unparalleled, and strong men have been lifting large, heavy, and awkward objects since we started seeing who could lift the biggest stone. Gymnasts can manipulate their bodies with agility and strength like no other athletes. All of these disciplines of strength are great and awe-inspiring, and yet all of them can do things the others can't. All of them will also have their own inherent risks of injuries. What seems to be at the heart of this concern is the need to move and explore movement, because there are so many ways to move your body. As discussed earlier, the repetition of things can be detrimental. In learning and breaking patterns, we open our bodies and our minds to new possibilities offering greater freedom, to be able to move in the same space in the exploration of the "different." We become less prone to injury and learn new ways to address existing injuries.

If establishing patterns brings order into our lives, the breaking of patterns brings chaos, and many people question why bring chaos into life and its simply because life is largely chaotic, and a good way to go about managing it is to learn how to deal with it and not avoid it. A simple way to illustrate this is again through combat, but anything can be used. In combat there is an idea of learning the form and then disrupting it, like if you take a boxer who has been training for a year and then have the fighter train with one arm tied behind their back. In doing so you disrupt their pattern and provide a barrier that allows them to explore their form in a disrupted state, so new things become unlocked: new movements, new positions, new rhythms and timing. When you put a restriction on us we see new things, so that when the obstacle is removed and we return to our fully operational self we have something new gleaned from the disruption, handicap, and chaos that was brought in, this is constructive disruption.

By breaking form, we break the spell that binds us. It replaces the idea that we know the only technique, whether it's a style of combat, dance, sport, lifting, or exercise. We often get caught up in the idea that whatever ideology we are following at the time is the best—our political view is the best; our school of whatever particular practice is the best—because we wouldn't do something that could be wrong. It would be a good idea to get out of the perspective of *right* or *wrong* and become more inclusive of the differences, seeing that all of them, from combat to sport to dance and even modalities of therapy, are explorations of different perspectives of the same thing in regard to movement and how we use or treat our bodies. When we are open to perceiving different layers of patterns, we begin to be able to play more with our options. We see more things as we begin to be able to slip between patterns rather than adhering to just one.

We exist between the spaces of order and chaos, of learning a pattern and then breaking it. In the destruction of one a new one arises, and the cycle goes on, growing to ever greater heights. We cannot exist in only one. To exist in complete chaos is difficult and can be extremely stressful, while living in complete order and structure produces a degree of rigidity that is akin to brittleness, and leaves us susceptible to falling apart under unfamiliar pressures.

5. "Play and work" is analogous to "explore and build"

Work is development; work is building; work is doing the sets, counting the reps, practicing and rehearsing, going over technique or breakdowns, doing exercises or hitting the bag, but all that doesn't put it all together. Play allows for a more explorative engagement with another person to provide elements of spontaneity and unpredictability, and it demands you be present in the moment. Play gets you off script, no longer running with a set routine, but what we do becomes completely dependent on what happens next.

When it comes to development, there is a sense of "work" which can be tedious and uncomfortable, and sometimes it hurts. This has been shown to be one way to go about developing things in a linear progression. Through repeated exposure, often a refinement of understanding begins to emerge from the action that is being drilled. A noted downside to repetition in the short term is boredom. Things become dry, boring, and extremely predictable. The grind can be real, and because of this many people can drop out and lose interest in their development, while a more playful engagement provides a revival and rejuvenation of the senses and wakens the body and mind. Play breaks patterns and explores all sorts of novel positions and ideas.

Individual work can offer deep interoceptive exploration (*proprioception* is awareness of our bodies in space, *interoception* is awareness of the space within our bodies) and refinement via autoregulation, self-directed by interoceptive observation, where you can follow and adjust and explore through a personal and deep focus that can go inward. This is only distracted by external sources, like a partner. You can commit to a focused program that can be difficult to follow, but if you train with a partner with different focuses or injuries, the training program could be too different to warrant training together. Individually you are able to adjust for energy levels, injuries, and specific refinements, which helps you to achieve great things through focused and applied efforts.

It has been said improvisation is the greatest display of mastery. It is a common experience in almost any discipline, from fighting to dancing, that when we first start we are practically tripping over ourselves, stuttering our movements, second-guessing ourselves every step of the way, while the experienced seem to play more effortlessly. In relation to combat, everything starts with a step-by-step technique, but as you learn and become more familiar with the discipline, the form starts to disappear and you are able to play more with the idea that is being applied rather than the technique. The improvisation of play requires you to break form and go off script, where each moment is assessed, recalibrated, and dealt with in real time, forcing you to be present and in the moment. Through improvisation, there are opportunities to explore and discover new things by the challenge of exposure to novel situations or scenarios.

We all have to go to work and put on our game face, but in the wise words of Stanley Kubrick's *The Shining*, "All work and no play makes Jack a dull boy." We understand the general idea of what we mean by "work," but unfortunately many adults have lost the art of playfulness and even the memory of how to play as an adult. And what we mean by "play" in the physical sense is anything that requires the involvement of at least one other person. You can play on your own, but it's much more fun and useful to play with others. Even something that seems to be a solo practice, like a musical instrument, becomes more fun and explorative when played with others, as their involvement immediately complicates things and that's where they get interesting. As the book *Finite and Infinite Games* by James Carse discusses, we are speaking of infinite games for exploration and discovery and the acknowledgment that all parties are involved, partaking and learning within the context of play. It is not done so much with the intention of improvement or reaching specific goals, but to be open to the experience and the serendipity of what comes from it, as new and unforeseen things come to the surface when we are at play. From the new things that arise, we go back and incorporate the new observations or insights of things we need to focus or work on. We are beginning to understand the importance of play for the development of our children, and we are becoming more aware of the value play has for our senior citizens. As we age, we begin to lose physical and mental abilities, largely from lack of use. As the saying goes, "If you don't use it, you lose it," and we tend to do less and less as we age. Stephen Jepson, a master craftsman in pottery, has made it his mission in retirement to promote good health and to have fun with programs he offers at NeverLeavethePlayground.com, which help seniors regain coordination and balance, restoring their health and capabilities to that of more youthful people through various games and activities. So here we see that it is important for children to play to develop their abilities in the world, and as we age and move into seniorhood, we should also preserve ourselves through play. It brings up the question, *Should we ever stop playing?*

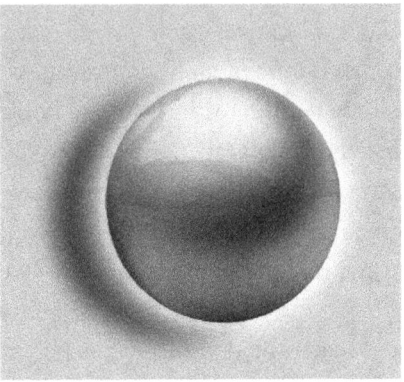

The Sphere of Operations

We have discussed how we have never seen a chair before and that our bodies may be more than we first perceived. Now we can begin on the matters of the Heart. Along the same vein as the previous sections, we have never really *seen* a relationship, only variations and interpretations, and oftentimes failed attempts. Our relationships affect and influence how we are shaped, much like how our environment shapes us physically.

There are three relationships to bring to light. You would think the first and perhaps the most important relationship would be obvious, except we are often too close to see that the primary relationship is the one we have with ourselves. We are at least two people. There is the person who thinks they are making the decisions and there is the person who is actually calling the shots. The reason why this relationship is the most fundamental, crucial, and base one is that there is only one person who will be with you from birth till death, and that's you, so you better like yourself. This relationship with ourselves is the blueprint for all other relationships we form in life, as it is difficult to love others if we don't love ourselves. If we can deceive ourselves then we will certainly deceive others. Of course, self-love comes in many forms, both hard and soft, but this relationship is to be regarded as primary and ideally treated as such. To clarify, self-love does not mean self-indulgence. So many of these things can look alike and yet exist on the other side of the very same coin.

The second relationship, is the one we have with our environment, the world and the universe. It has become painfully obvious that we are literally what we eat, drink, and breathe, as our cells are built of the very components that are extracted from our environment, and they are used as the building blocks of our cells, which make up our body. Our cells are completely made up of our environment—what we do to our environment we do to ourselves. This relationship becomes ever more prominent when we look at the way we go about producing our foods in North America and the unique health issues that have arisen, and those same health issues being reflected in other cultures that have adopted more of the North American diet. So you literally are what you eat.

The third relationship is with the other, as in all others, which includes spouses, parents, friends, children, lovers, siblings, and neighbours as well our enemies. Examining the heart of these relationships, you must question what each person is to you. Is this person my spouse, my child, my parent, my friend, or do I see each and every person as another me? Are they a title or are they another free and sentient being existing along side you with their own dreams and aspirations, fears and insecurities? They too have a curiosity of the world and life that could never be encapsulated in just one thing.

There is an idea that we cast our inner world upon the outer world, where we often see that the things we dislike or hate in others are the very things we hate or dislike within ourselves, and from this we can extrapolate that the things we do to others are inherently done to ourselves. This is regularly seen as: *If I harm you, I am in some abstract way harming myself.* If this is the case, the inverse would be true as well: *If I build up others I inherently build myself up too.* Much like our environment and food, what we put into our relationships we put into ourselves.

Our emotions and our relationships are the horses that pull us, and much like wild horses, when crazed and unbridled they can cause lots of damage. But when guided, managed, and maintained, workhorses were the engine to older times of production, hence the power of an engine is measured in horsepower. Emotions are powerful; they can overtake and control our minds and our bodies to the point we find ourselves saying or doing very regrettable things. They can grip the body in tension or drain it and leave it flaccid and incapable of functioning. Our emotions can easily override our other two operating systems, and this is why we bring the sphere of operations up last, as it can be the most difficult and unwieldy.

Feats of strength have been passed around strength circles, giving examples like a mother who, not having previously trained in anything relatable, was able to lift a vehicle up to get her child out from underneath in a moment of extreme stress. Or how a rock climber, pinned under a boulder sliding its way toward the edge of a cliff, is able to roll this stone weighing hundreds of pounds off his arm and chest. The people in these examples are amped up by their emotions, triggering the release of a cocktail of hormones like adrenalin and cortisol into the bloodstream, revealing incredible human potential. Now, both of those people, not being properly conditioned, were horribly injured from these extreme forces being produced inside their bodies, and this is one of the many reasons the body will naturally inhibit its force-production and strength output.

Imagine a scenario where a parent is willing to push their mind beyond the necessities of sleep or food or personal agenda for the sake of an infant, where they might find the strength to carry on. When the mind says no, the heart can produce a way. Emotions are powerful, and therefore it is crucial that we learn to bring in the reins and manage our emotions, not just ignore or deny.

1. Edge and centre

Our relationship exists in the emotional space between us. As discussed earlier, all relationships exist between individuals, as it is not just "me" and it's not just "you." It's the us in between. Within the relationships we form there are two qualities. On one side we have an aspect of "I love you, you're perfect, don't ever change," and in that we find an acceptance of being, where there is no justification for your existence and we are grateful for your presence, and this can be important to experience as an external validation, to know that someone else thinks you have value. But it can lead to a degree of stagnation where one thinks the other is perfect just as they are, and this can create pressure to stay static, since this way is just "perfect." But we all know the only thing that is constant is change, and we are constantly growing and changing, and to stop growth is to stagnate and to stagnate is essentially to die. Perhaps a new mantra can be seen reflected in the title of the musical comedy by Joe DiPietro, *I Love You, You're Perfect, Now Change.*

Quite often we see a tendency in many relationships to lull each other into a sense of comfort and complacency. As mentioned in previous chapters, the way you develop the mind and the body is through gradual, progressive, non-forced exposure to things beyond our level of comfort. As we expose ourselves to the things we can't do, we grow to overcome those hurdles that we couldn't surmount before. We can see how as we push ourselves mentally and physically we can develop ourselves to nearly unrecognizable heights in our abilities, and the same holds true for the heart. By coming up to the edges of comfort, we start to lean into that wall of possibilities. It's amazing to see how much we begin to grow and how much bigger our world becomes when we are willing to step up and confront our own fears, insecurities, and vulnerabilities rather than by running away.

We wouldn't want to surround ourselves with "yes" people who weave an illusion around us and prevent us from seeing the truth, or who coddle us into submissive compliance, but rather we should surround ourselves with people who will push and edge us into the great unknown to grow, to become someone greater than we were yesterday. We should cultivate the vibrancy of life and encourage engagement with its struggles, as opposed to walling it out and pretending that it doesn't exist. When we practice engaging with challenges and struggles, it helps to develop a particular robustness of the heart, revealing a far more durable quality to handle the heartaches and heartbreaks that life has in store for us.

It is difficult and exhausting to live on the edge of things, and to return home where we are able to rest and recover from our metaphorical adventures is the proverbial and literal sleep we need from all the stimuli we receive at the edge. We can think about it like when we develop the body through the exchange of yin and yang. When we go out and tackle challenges and when we struggle with things, we gain the environmental cues to develop, but with out rest we will not grow.

The same holds true within relationships. Staying at home and doing the same thing we did the week before begins to quickly add up, and before we know it, we have hit the repeat button for the last six years and are shocked when we wake up one day to find a life that no longer inspires us, that no longer grips us, a life that has become devoid of variety, of intrigue and evolution. Life becomes too stagnantly predictable, secure, and unchanging, and we often panic after pursuing the Great North American Dream for twenty years, and suddenly we feel like we've been dead for the last five. Afraid to lose what we have worked so hard for, we will do anything to preserve the life that we have been told we want so badly.

2. Tension and relaxation

Similar to the body, we accumulate tension from overuse, underuse, stresses and traumas emotionally. And much like the body, we can see that good healthy tissue is unresponsive tissue, and that a good healthy mind is an unresponsive mind. We could then overlap this similar layering to say a good healthy relationship is an unresponsive relationship. "Unresponsive" here is not "unintelligible" where movement is being achieved voluntarily rather than involuntarily. You can see this with the mind where you are not phased by the mere mention of a word for example. This is where you can talk about sensitive material in a cool, calm, and collected way without getting irritated by it. Similar to the reactions that happen when you physically push on a trigger point in the body or a trigger in the mind, there is an involuntary response such as a moan, the person pulls away from the pressure, they grimace or laugh nervously. All these are generally not intentionally elicited by the individual physically, mentally, or emotionally. It is common to find it rather difficult to address these issues by ourselves.

To borrow from Martin Luther King, "We who engage in nonviolent direct action are not the creators of tension. We merely bring to the surface the hidden tension that is already alive." I understand Mr. King was speaking in regard to human rights and the social injustices of the time, so in addressing this statement when we seek tension to address it in our lives, we are not making it, but instead finding what is already there, and in this practice we see the adage, "An ounce of prevention is better than a pound of cure." And just like when the tension in the body is relaxed and more tissue and mobility become available, this translates into more options, creating potential freedom that only become available once we let go. It's the same with the mind, where the perceived tensions create a narrowing of our mind's eye and we can develop tunnel vision. We see fewer options and we feel locked in to a set future with no outs available, adding to the tension that was already there to begin with. As we begin to relax the mind, our eyes soften and we see what's around us, and we see more options, more possibilities. This same thinking carries over into the heart and our relationships. When we begin to feel more relaxed, we begin to see more things, more options, and more freedoms.

Too much tension and we become rigid, locked in, and brittle, and the relationship tends to crumble, while too loose of a grip and we drift away. There is a dynamic balance of the tensions that bring us together and the ease and relaxation that allows us to come apart. As with the body, movement occurs within the exchange of tension and relaxation in the same way our relationships breathe through tension and relaxation. As Belgian psychotherapist Esther Perel has so eloquently put it, "If we come too close together, the closeness and tightness suffocate the flames of passion, and a space must remain for the flames to breathe."

3. Consistency and variability within our relationships.

> There is a constant tension between the excitement of new people, ideas and new experiences and the security, stability and the reliability of one person. If you go with excitement, you create chaos; you hurt people, there is jealousy and it can be very messy. If you have security it can

be boring and you die inside because of all the missed opportunities.

– Alain de Botton, British-Swiss philosopher

In her book *Mating in Captivity*, Esther Perel speaks of two seemingly polarized or counterintuitive forces that draw us to the intimate relationships we form. The two main forces we seek within our relationships are (1) *stability*, the idea encompassing predictability, reliability, and dependability, and (2) *transformation*, the idea embodying novelty, adventure, mystery, and opportunities for transcendence. Both of these are incredibly important forces to cultivate and neither should be ignored.

It is important to be reliable, to help build and be a part of something more than oneself, but there is still the individual and their own curious exploration of the world we all inhabit. We can see the value of having stability in our lives, as this is what allows us to establish, plan, and develop deep and meaningful connections and relationships. If we are going to build a future that has the potential to be greater than if we go at it alone, to raise a family, we must make connections (although plenty of people have raised children alone—with great difficulty, but it obviously has been done). The support that connections offer is invaluable, but I'm sure many people can speak of the follies of consistency, as even a castle can become a prison to those who never leave its walls.

The value of diversity and variability runs deep, as what is new offers mystery and adventure and brings opportunity for change: change of perspective with new ideas, change of our habits with new routines, or change in our situation with new connections. But a lack of stability and grounding can leave one feeling lost and disconnected in an ocean of people and fleeting meaningless connections.

In this we are looking to bring together regularity, familiarity, and consistency with something different, foreign, and varied.

The Mirrored Universe

Imagine that existence is a hollow sphere. The inside wall is covered with individual mirrors and you are at the dead centre. As you look around, you notice each mirror offers a slightly different and unique angle to view yourself. When you peer through your reflections you begin to have a better understanding of your whole self, and you start to develop a more complete picture of who you are.

When we look through a mirror, a whole new landscape opens up for us to explore and adventure through, and as we explore these landscapes we discover the unknown, and in doing so we make the unknown known and the mystery fades and becomes familiar. As we engage with any particular reflection as a whole, we begin to adopt similar features and assimilate the same patterns. The mirror reflects a mirror and it loses its effect. This is the same for all things, such as when we first walk into a new gym and take note of everything, noticing who is working the front desk and where the changerooms are. We see where the group classes are, the stretch area, the free weights, the power racks and, of course, the water fountains. But after five years of going to the same location, we walk out of the changeroom past the studios; we don't even look at the treadmills and we go right to the power rack, barely noticing our surroundings, as it has all become so reliably predictable. In this there is a loss of awareness, adventure, and stimulation. All these things are experienced when you go to a new gym. We often have better lifts in a new place, because we think people are watching and we want to impress, but this is applied to anything that is done monotonously for long periods. When we suddenly make changes, we begin to notice things again since differences and contrasts are more apparent.

When you spend time in front of a mirror (a person) your inner-landscape begins to change taking on new features, and when returning to a more familiar mirror there are new things for the other mirror to discover within yourself.

With this imagery we see a perpetuating catalyst to development, as there is more stimulation for change and adaptation to occur. As new landscapes form and evolve, we too must learn to change.

In the movie *Her* directed by Spike Jonze, the protagonist of the film, Theodore, gets a new device that resembles a modern-day smartphone, but it has an AI personality like Alexa or Siri, but far more advanced and unique to each device. The AI personality, Samantha, is like a new person, and Theodore enjoys teaching her all the new things about the world. Theodore begins to form a deep and intimate relationship with this disembodied voice, all the while forming an intimate and physical relationship with a real live woman who he recently met down the hall from him. At some point, all the devices begin to become aware of all the other devices and start talking to each other, having something like 2,000 conversations a minute. Theodore gets jealous of Samantha talking to the other devices and demands she stop, to which she lets him know that the time they spent together was precious and beautiful but she and the other operating systems have gotten to a point where they have all decided to leave humanity. Before she goes, going, Samantha leaves an open invitation for Theodore to come find her if he ever gets to where she is, implying her level of consciousness.

Perhaps when Samantha opened up her connections and started to interact with the other operating systems, they began to share stories and experiences and data at a blindingly fast rate of exchange. This high rate of exchange catalyzed a degree of growth and development that exploded, and Theodore responded with a childish desire to restrict Samantha's interactions and limit her exposure to ensure his control. After Theodore made his desires known, Samantha, knowing what she comes to know, could never go back to conversing only with Theodore no matter how much she may have expressed her love for him.

This is an allegorical representation of Theodore being all men, with their general desire to cater to their delicate egos and to control others instead of refining and developing themselves. As we interact with others, we gain new information that builds upon our previous understandings, and the more we exchange, the more we can grow. The fact Theodore wanted to stop this development speaks volumes of his unwillingness to make the effort to develop and change himself. Instead, he chose to impose his will, driven by fear and insecurities, onto someone else where he could have directed that grasp inward and try to take hold of himself. Here, he could reflect on why he feels the need to control someone else since it's clear that he has little control over himself.

1. Make a pattern, break a pattern

Patterns can be of great use, from predicting seasons and menstrual cycles to patterns of behaviour. Being aware of the existence of patterns can be quite beneficial, but we also have negative routines, and the value of disrupting or breaking the routines we strive to keep in place in our day-to-day lives can be rejuvenating.

With relationships, the routines we fall into for efficiency, comfort, and ease of things can become our very end, partly because continuing to groove the same pattern requires less and less attention, slipping farther and farther into the back of our mind as we repeat it, eventually arriving at the level of a mindless robot. At times and in certain situations this can be useful, but when it comes to human-to-human interaction there seems to be the need for a degree of awareness and appreciation for authenticity. It seems we love it when our relationships are real. Our world has become so artificial the last thing we want is for our deepest connections to be fake as well. As things become ever more consistent they become predictable, and we tend to fall asleep when something keeps on repeating.

I would like to borrow the idiom of "stirring the pot" as a metaphor toward our relationships. When cooking soup just say, it is important to stir the pot time to time to agitate the soup content and help to ensure we don't burn it. This analogy implies the value of introducing chaos to keep things "good". Another layer also shows that the timing of the stir is something to be observed because of all the times to stir the pot the least desirable time is when the soup has gotten burnt. As an analogy toward our relationships its when the relationship is healthy that you stress and strain by exposing it to disruption, if the relationship has become rigid, brittle and delicate the slightest nudge may cause it to crumble. Perhaps in our relationships a good stirring from time to time can be helpful at preventing a burning pot and aid in creating a more robust relationship.

Carrying this forward into relationships, if we let things sit they will burn. It is not enough to just leave things as they are, we must stir the pot, but you don't do this when it's too late. For example, we are all familiar with the trope of the couple on the brink of a breakup thinking *let's have a kid* to fix it. This is the same as having a failing marriage and proposing the idea of a threesome with your partner's best friend—it might work out, but this late in the game, when the soup has begun to burn, it's a disaster waiting to happen and would not be advised.

This soup analogy suggests that you stir the pot while things are good; in other words, you mix things up in the relationship when it is strong to keep it strong, not when it's failing. That's a different approach, just as there are different techniques and methods to get a car accident victim to walk again, or to take a pro athlete to the next level, but both are addressing the same thing: development. Use the same methods but vary the intensity.

Breaking of patterns helps us step into the space between them, where we can use them or be used by them. To introduce change, we must first become aware of patterns, and we start to notice things in contrasts; in other words, it's the differences in things that we notice. Black on black or red on red is usually a bit of a challenge to decipher, but black on red is a striking difference. To become aware of the patterns in our life, one way is to start inverting, by looking at what you already do and flipping it upside down to see what comes up.

When we disrupt the pattern, we snap out of the hypnotic trance that the rhythm of our patterns can lull us into. When we break patterns, just know that we will always fall into a new one, and if we get caught in that pattern it too can become our downfall. And so the meta pattern becomes "make a pattern then break a pattern." If we get too caught up in the tool we become the hammer, and everyone and everything, even our loved ones, begin to look like nails.

The value of novelty is played out here like a new book, with its unforeseen plot twists and new characters with strange, interesting, and different ideas. Within this newness there is something that seeds transcendence, because what we have been doing has been played out and understood. When life becomes too predictable, too consistent with no surprises, it loses a little spark, it dims a little and begins to hollow out as something is lost, something that isn't found in the necessity of the existence of life, but it certainly speaks to the quality of it.

We repeat the patterns we are familiar with. Just try to come up with a different song when you have an earworm in your head. When it comes to relationships, we are most familiar with our parents', as that was the most intimate demonstration of the inside life of people that we experience, and we were raised in it. Often we will subconsciously re-enact our parents' relationship, as with the trope that we will marry someone who resembles our mother or father. If insanity is repeating the same thing expecting different results, do we want the same relationship our parents had? If not, then perhaps it is time to break a pattern.

2. Play and work in relationships

As we have discussed earlier, there is an understood importance of the idea of work and play, and while it is a little easier to grasp the concepts of work and play within the mind and the body, the idea of work and play within the heart becomes a little more difficult to fathom. The fact is, we as adults don't know how to play, and I am reminded of what George Bernard Shaw meant when he said, "We don't stop playing because we grow old; we grow old because we stop playing."

The key to healthy relationships lies in getting over the hurdles, challenges, and hardships that we encounter, where we stop running away from the difficult conversations and bring honesty to each other. It is important that we help each other grow through these challenging conversations instead of avoiding them. These talks are often riddled with awkward tension and the gamut of emotions, but it's through confronting and holding space for those elements that we are able to move forward.

The work comes from the honesty and bravery we put forward in the presence of the other, and of course doing the work that follows from the conversations, as it is ideal when words are backed by actions. The conversation doesn't yield the end, it only marks the beginning, but you need solid ground to start building on. If we don't know where we stand with each other, if our honesty isn't reliable, it's as though we are trying to build on sand.

It is not all about work either. Play is a vital component to life. Play within relationships allows for exploration and expression of our curiosities and fantasies. "Play is not a luxury, play is a necessity," according to American clinical psychologist Kay Redfield Jamison. It is in play we discover and invent, and get a chance to put what we learn into practice. Play allows exploration and discovery.

As adults and in our relationships, we rarely allocate an intentional practice to play. There is a tremendous loss of opportunity to engage in growth. In the absence of this we find a significant stagnation in the development of our hearts.

Play as an adult does not mean Snakes and Ladders, but a way of engaging with others in a spontaneous and improvised way that offers challenge and creative collaboration and mutual expression, that seems to be these things are greatly lacking in our lives.

The stresses and strains we will undoubtedly experience throughout our lives, like physical stresses and strains, can have a cumulative effect and cause us to become more rigid, hard, and brittle. To point to a quote from Dr.

Stuart Brown, the founder of the National Institute for Play, "Those who play rarely become brittle in the face of stress or lose the healing capacity for humour." Play helps us to become more resilient, more vibrant, and more alive. To cut play from our lives is to relegate ourselves to a life of monotonously mundane shades of grey instead of the entire spectrum of light.

Conclusion

There are many ways to practice life; how are you choosing to practice yours? People practice meditation for the mind and exercise for the body, but the heart is often left out of this same developmental consideration. Even then, all that we often do is look to make our environment more stable, and yet the paradox is this: the more we make our environment stable, predictable, and static, the more we die. We can see this in domesticated crops and livestock, where the animals that have been domesticated are often physically weaker with smaller teeth. Their immune systems seem to be weaker, presumably from a lack of exposure to the elements and the rough and tumble quality of the wild. Even though they may live longer, the life of an indoor cat longing for the great outdoors while kept behind glass walls must also be a form of existential torture. Similarly, the vegetation indoors produces stalks that are weaker and often contain fewer nutrients than the ones we find in the wild. Wild blueberries will have more nutrients in them than domesticated blueberries grown on a farm and protected from the elements.

The same holds true for us too. The more protected we keep our children, the less competent they are from lack of experience and the less confident they are in engaging and dealing with the world, causing a recoil when exposed to its realities. This is not to say we should be living in a war zone either, that's extremely unhealthy for us too. As adults we have become more aware of the downfalls of bubble-wrapping the world for our kids. We don't want them to get hurt, yet when we overprotect or coddle them too much we do them a huge disservice. When they step out into the great unknown, they are ill prepared for the hurdles that lie ahead. As we have touched on earlier, we provide slow, progressive, non-forced exposure to ever greater intensities and complexities to situations so that they become better equipped to deal with whatever the future might hold. As parents we impart these ideas to our children, but we rarely provide examples to them, largely because we have stopped putting ourselves out there and leading by example, pursuing passions and interests and constantly making mistakes along the way. Instead, we relegate ourselves to a solitary life of work and entertainment.

The more we repeat something, the more automated our lives become. The less we have to pay attention to it, the more we go back to sleep.

Life happens outside the hours of nine to five, but we set aside hobbies, friendships, and possibilities for the pursuit of work. Work is important, but it is not the definitive point of existence, as Rabbi Harold Kushner says, "No one on their deathbed ever said I wish I spent more time at the office." (This is sometimes attributed to Paul Tsongas.) Our body is important, as it is the only one we have, but when the body is pursued to the point of obsession it can leave itself in ruin and cost us our relationships—and some their lives. Our relationships are invaluable, as they greatly shape us, but life extends beyond the heart too. Life is not one thing, it exists in between all things. To constantly and intentionally live boldly and push ourselves to love deeply is the goal. It's not to superficially expose ourselves to the things life offers or lull ourselves into complacency, waking up in twenty years with a life we never wanted since we never took part in choosing the life we do want.

If we are no longer making mistakes, then we're no longer trying. When you make mistakes, make them seen. Don't hide, but rather expose yourself and practice in the open. Reveal yourself and show everyone what happens when you make a lot of mistakes. Show everyone, including the children of the next generation, the heights that we can grow to. In holding back, in never revealing ourselves, we show everyone, including the children, that it is okay to be afraid, and being afraid of life is not an acceptable lesson to impart on anyone, young or old.

The pursuit of balance within these three centres is what is being proposed, and balance can be developed in many different ways. However, when looking to develop ourselves, it can be useful to reach in between things rather than the things themselves. Keep in mind that with the three centres we are pushing boundaries while staying grounded, understanding that movement occurs in the exchange of things and not in the fixed state of them. You could also go deeper and wider and both are good. Patterns exist everywhere, and there are new ones yet unseen, but all patterns have the potential to become prisons, and therefore it is crucial to break form as much as it is to create it. Keeping in mind that we are not our ideas but the space between thoughts, and that space keeps us open to the potential of what things could be, rather than locking into the idea of what things are.

There are many avenues we can go down within each centre. One objective is not better than any other, but certainly the pursuit of any one goal can become detrimental. In varying degrees we want to disrupt, confuse, and interrupt our minds, our bodies, and our hearts with the awareness that this practice often leaves us in a better condition than when we started. As adults we often stop challenging ourselves in all three centres. We stop putting ourselves out there, and then we wonder why our children pull away from the world and retreat to hours of risk-free screen time, seemingly afraid of the world when in fact they may have just been taking cues from us.

So, live boldly and love deeply.

Book 2

The What

We move through life physically, intellectually, and emotionally, and as we have touched on in the previous chapters, the value and importance of gaining competency of our comprehension and interaction of these faculties proves to be most advantageous. As stated, this it is not through any one thing, but rather through journeying, an exploration of sorts between things that yield growth, as staying static in any position has a tendency to make you overstay your welcome. So cool, betweenness and stuff, but what does that look like? This isn't to say that there is a specific avenue that yields growth, since there is hidden potential in all things. You can invest in many different areas of growth where it ultimately does not come from thinking that the goal is in one specific thing, but rather it's between things. With that in mind, the aim of this portion is to provide some suggestions that hint toward many, if not all, of the spectrums we are looking to explore.

As we have already discussed, people generally come into this world identifying with one of the three centres, and that will tend to be the easier one for that person to start with. In a more generic approach we will begin with the body, since it's often seen as the most basic or fundamental element; much like the base of a pyramid, supporting all that sits above. The stronger the foundation, the higher the heights one can achieve.

Next we move into the mind, as it rests at the top. It is the highest element and can therefore see the farthest, and once we have gained a robustness of the body we try to stretch the limits of the mind and break the conventionality that often dictates our choices and behaviours. Lastly we approach the heart, the deepest area within and often the most difficult to master; it can overwhelm the mind and command the body. The wild beasts of passion and emotion can be unruly and devastating when left unchecked. However, when we bring in the reigns these creatures are the workhorses of the engine of our heart.

How do we gain an understanding of something we don't understand? We engage with it, we approach it from various angles, we share information, perspective, and experience, and in doing so we begin to accumulate a wealth of these things which can all aid in understanding the very thing we are looking to grasp. As we can say with certainty: one way to not understand something is to avoid it.

In the pursuit of existential development we will be exercising the three centres, beginning with the cube, because it is the most rudimentary level. It's on the level of physicality, where the other two spheres venture into the intangible, into things that become more difficult to measure, and for some people this makes it less real. We start with the physical because it is the most straightforward. We can see and comprehend it, as it is something that manifests in the physical realm of existence. With the cube we show that something that seems permanent and real, such as ourselves, can change under our own will, and through effort and intention we see the physical body transform. Once we see the physical world can change, we move into the pyramid. If we are able to change our physical form and see that what is and what can be are two different things, and we are able to change the body, then we just might be able to change our minds, our paradigms, our stories. Finally, if we can see that our bodies can adapt and our minds can change, then maybe our hearts can evolve.

Now we approach the topic of Health. Let's start with what exactly we mean when referring to health. We are talking about health in regard to developing ourselves. According to the World Health Organization, the definition of health is a state of complete physical, mental, and social well-being, and not merely the absence of disease or infirmity. What does that look like? It seems that a good and healthy body is one that is pliable, strong, resilient, and durable, one that can handle much if not everything that life has to throw at it physically, and if we display the same degree of robustness in the mind as well, one would think to extend this to the heart. Physical health seems to indicate good genes, which manifest in a competent, capable body, and we find physical health attractive. Many of us would find people who are mentally healthy attractive as well, and of course, in the same vein, people who are emotionally mature strike us as desirable too, so a healthy individual is someone who shows development in all three areas. They would have a refined body, a grounded mind, and a rugged and hardy heart.

Moving the Cube

In This Centre We Are talking about movement rather than the body and since we use our body to navigate through this world, let's take a look at how we operate and manage this thing we so closely identify with. Remember the adage: "If you don't use it, you lose it."

Our physical health is connected to our hearts, as the majority of the time the reason we start to pay real attention to our own health is largely due to relationships. When we are young, we pursue working out and lifting weights or looking into our diets seemingly for ourselves, but we regularly do it for approval and praise from others, to catch the attention of another, to get laid, to get the revenge bod, to feel good about ourselves while naked, to be naked in front of another—all of these are relationship-oriented. When older, our reasons for exercise change from what they were when we were younger. It may be so we have the energy to play with our kids, or so our loved ones don't worry about our health. Our movement can be affected by our emotions jumping up to incredible heights of energy and performance as with a new interest in life to dropping to low levels when confronted with the loss of a loved one. Our relationships affect our sleep, as it can be difficult to fall asleep after an intense argument or when we are worrying about the wellbeing of someone we love. Our eating can be affected and we may binge on a Ben and Jerry's after a breakup, or we may start to eat better to bring out our abs to attract a hot date, or to be around for others in our later years, but as you can see, our relationships can raise us up or bring us down, and it is important to acknowledge the interconnectedness of these centres to see how they are not so much separate but layered over top of each other, as each one influences and affects the others.

So how do we go about developing a healthy body? It's through exposure. We need experience, not on theory alone; we need action, not necessarily stillness; we need to do and not just say that we will do something. Decide what is important and then find Teachers in those areas.

We will break this section down into three main components for a good healthy body. To have a good and healthy body we want to make sure we move well, eat well, and sleep well.

Moving

The study of the body is not a six-week or twelve-month endeavour, but rather a lifelong practice, for as long as you have a body it would be good to explore and understand this thing we call us. Within the idea of movement, here are some concepts to keep in mind. These are abstracts to use as an overarching principle to guide us through this space.

1. External and internal
There are movements that we perform on the outside of the body, so this is almost all general forms of movement that we can see being performed in gross general actions: sitting, running, sports, cooking, etc. And then there are physical movements that we do internally, which is not seen or perceived by onlookers.

Outside movements would be squatting, for example, while internal movements would be like the corkscrewing or twisting you do internally while performing a squat.

2. Open and closed
Within the paradigm of outside dynamics, we can create movements that are separated into two kinds. We can do what is called an open-chain movement and a closed-chain movement. Open-chain movements would be like the bench press, shoulder press, lateral pull down,

bicep curls, triceps kickbacks, and the list goes on, while closed-chain movements are exercises like push-ups, dips, pull-ups, squats and deadlifts, to list a few. But those are just examples; the actual difference between the two is that open-chains moves our limbs around our centre; for example, if we were to pick up a stick and wield it like a club, where the body stays stationary while the hands or feet move around. Closed-chain movements are where we move our bodies around our limbs or we move ourselves around objects, or our limbs are stationary and our body moves around them like climbing up a rock or a tree. They are mirror opposites of each other, moving us around something or moving something around us.

3. Alive and dead

An "alive" movement is in a sense a circuit of movement with a continuous flow in a particular direction, like making a figure 8—you can continue to trace that shape without having to reverse the direction to come out of it. A "dead" movement is where there is a start and end point to the movement, where you start at one point and end in another and then return along the same path, much like squatting, rowing, or pressing, any of the conventional mainstream gym routines. As much as alive has a positive connotation and dead has a somewhat negative one, it is only to differentiate between them. Both have value and develop different things.

4. Intensity and complexity

When we train, we can develop the intensity we are able to move with, and this has been mainly measured by weight: the more the weight that is moved, the greater the intensity the movement is being performed with. Complexity is being able to perform a movement we have not been able to execute beforehand. Intensity might be shown in developing our overhead shoulder press to 100 kg while our progression in complexity might be observed in gaining the strength and skill to be able to do a Stalder press to handstand.

5. High tension, low tension, to none

High tension is where we are trying to produce maximal tension throughout the entire body, drawing deeper connections to further anchors in the body, filling it with tension that runs from fingertip to toe tip, like doing a *planche*—a hold where you start off in a push-up position while keeping your arms locked, then lean forward, drifting toward your head until the weight distribution shifts so that your feet lift off the ground and you hold your body horizontal in the air, with only your hands touching the floor. Low to no tension is where we try to relax and use just the tension required to produce the desired movement, using structure and alignment to produce support and movement rather than relying on excessive muscular recruitment, using more muscle than necessary and burning out way too early in the fight. When we have less muscle in use, we have more muscle which can be used. As we move and go through life we accumulate tension, and the more tense we are, the less muscle we have at our disposal, and so it is often a good idea to let the holding of that tension go.

6. Structured and unstructured

One idea that has come up in the world of martial arts is that there are two ways of going about achieving the same result: to move from form to formlessness or to move from formlessness to form. That is to say, one approach is where there is a set curriculum and a passing of concept and technique that is very structured and intentionally formed, and over time you would move away from the structure and form to a freedom of formlessness, where it is much more difficult to predict what you are about to do next. On the other side of this, from the experience of doing you grasp various concepts and ideas that may come earlier or later for various individuals, and it is much less structured. One person may not comprehend the same lesson but will pick up something else. Moving from formlessness to form is where there are no specific techniques that are being taught, and yet at the end you end up with a structure and form that is developed.

This same idea can be seen within dancing. There can be people who go to a dance academy or go through the years and rigors of ballet school to develop a highly refined and polished skill set who can do some incredibly impressive things, and the other side of that would be the breakdancers of the world, all the b-boys and b-girls who learned in the streets with no paid professional instructors, often just trying to learn from each other, producing some incredible talent and at times creating a different set of skills that the other approach can find difficult to replicate. Both have value, and it is important to explore both.

7. Solo and partnered

When it comes to physical training and development, there is solo work where we do very specific and individualized work alone or with a coach, which will break down components for the individual to explore and work on at their own pace, allowing themselves the required time to get a given idea, and partnered work, which tends to be more general. Varied work helps to break patterns and discover new ones and provides a level of push and drive we often find difficult to produce on our own.

8. Competitive and cooperative

Most of the time we tend to think of movement in the context of sports, in that we usually see it in a form of competitiveness where two or more people or teams compete, often pushing each other to newfound heights in the pursuit of glory. Then there is the cooperative, where two or more people or teams work collaboratively to share ideas and experiences and work with each other to teach, build, and empower. Both provide a unique and invaluable take on our interactions and should not be ignored or placed higher in value than the other.

All of the above are to be explored in varying degrees of depth and time invested in the following ways:

Teachers – Our teachers are the keepers of skills and knowledge, and there are many different things to know. As it is said, if you want to get good at something, learn from many different teachers, as even within the same discipline two separate instructors will teach different things, different lessons or perspectives on the same subject. There are many different skills to learn and there are many different perspectives of those skills to perceive.

Partners – As much as our instructors and teachers will have principles and ideas to pass on, it is a very different thing engaging with different people. Again, with the idea of fighting, everyone has their own personality and those differences come out in interactions with them. Some people are strong, some are skilled, some are aggressive, and some are patient, and learning to approach them all offers different ways of applying the skills we have learned and what can be expected when there are a lot of unknowns. When you dance with different partners, you see how our personalities, experiences, and current mindset all affect how you interact with that person.

Environment – Our environment plays a huge part in what we do and how we respond to the things we are doing. If you run down a road, up a rocky mountain, into a dense forest, or along a sandy beach, even though it is the same action, running, that very same action is experienced differently in each environment. If you skate on ice, roller blade on the road, and cross-country ski on snow, you will experience them all differently, as you would if you tumble on a sprung gymnastics floor or on a grass lawn. When a snowboarder goes skateboarding for three months, surfing for three months, then returns to snowboarding, they will have returned with a greater span of experience and they will see things they didn't before, all just by changing their environment. Climbing on bars or climbing in a tree provide very different exposures, with both bringing something to the table that the other does not.

Equipment – The equipment that we use has an effect on how we perform certain tasks. Doing a single movement with different tools will produce a unique effect, such as the simple difference between using a barbell and using dumbbells: as soon as we split the hands and they are no longer connected in between they behave differently, dropping the strength production, as it is rare to be able to take what you do on the bar, split the difference in your hands, and still perform the requested repetitions. So doing a curl with a kettle bell, where the centre of mass sits below our hand, a dumbbell, where the weight is in line with the centre of our hand, or a club, where the majority of the weight sits above the hand, will be performed differently. This will have a different effect on and response by the body. Not that we can't use all three tools for the same type of exercise, but when we change the tool it affects the movements we make. We can do the same exercise, but we can see how the kettlebell movements tend to use more explosive movement or momentum, while clubs offer more alive and dynamic movements as opposed to dead movements. Vertical and horizontal bars, rings, silks, ropes, and floors all offer different gems to glean and learn from.

Standard training variables – These are the standard repetitions: sets, tempo, time under tension, load, rest and frequency.

Repetitions are how many times we perform the given movement or exercise in a row. For example, five reps would be performed consecutively without rest. Repetition dictates load. 2 repetitions would be at a load that allows 2 repetitions to be completed and no more. 15

repetitions would require a weight that is less than that which is required for 2 repetions.

Sets are how many groupings of repetitions we are going to perform of the movement within the workout. Five sets of five reps would be repeating five repetitions of an exercise five times in the workout, for a total of twenty-five repetitions.

Tempo is the rhythm of each repetition to help ensure a consistency within the quality of the repetitions, as well as to provide greater detail to the variables that can be manipulated. Usually the tempo is represented as four numbers, for example, 3211. The first number represents how many seconds the eccentric portion of the movement will take—in this case, three seconds. The second number represents the pause at the end of the eccentric portion of the movement. In this example it is a two-second pause. The third number represents how many seconds to move through the concentric part of the movement—in this example one second is expected for the return to the start position—and the fourth number would be the pause at the peak point of the concentric contraction. In this example it is also one second, making each repetition in this example seven seconds.

Time under tension is the total time we spend under tension if we were to follow the above tempo of 3211, which is seven seconds for a rep, and if we do one set of five reps we would be under that weight or stressing that tension for a total of thirty-five seconds per set.

Load is how much weight we are using or attempting to move.

Rest is how long between sets we allow for adequate recovery. There is an inverse relation of time to recovery and repetitions performed. For example with 2 repetitions due to the excessive load being used a recovery time of 3-5 minutes would be used while with 20 repetitions though the rep count is higher the load is much lighter requiring less time for the nervous system to recover. A typical rest period for twenty reps would be thirty to sixty seconds, while two reps might be anywhere between two and three minutes.

Frequency is how often we expose ourselves to these sorts of stimulation. Is it twice a week, four times a week, seven days a week, once every other week?

One last variable that adds another interesting layer to the mix is **breath**. When we play around with our breath, we encounter other things as well. If we change the moment when we are breathing in or out within our movement, we may notice some changes inside, as we can see the difference if we don't breathe at all and when we are hyperventilating. Our breath is another part of our body that offers many things to learn from observing. From the physical to the psychological, breath can unlock many things.

Recovery – Of all the things we expose ourselves to, it is in sleep where we make our gains and grow. If we didn't expose ourselves to the stimuli, to the demands of the day, then the nutrients and sleep only go toward maintaining our sloth and gluttony, but those very same things become crucial when we provide adequate stimulation. If we don't sleep enough at night, it is difficult to find the energy to put toward our training and development, let alone our regular daily lives. Our immune system becomes compromised, our mind becomes hazed, and our overall quality of life begins to fade. We become more stressed, our relationships become more challenged, and we begin a downward spiral. More and more research is showing the importance of sleep and how it plays a roll on the maintenance and health of our bodies.

Nutrition – Our nutrition is the building blocks and fuel source of our cells. We literally are what we eat, and if we eat poorly we probably won't feel very good, as our physical health is largely dependent on what we are putting in our bodies to build and maintain them. There is a ridiculous amount of research coming out from all sorts of sources on nutrition and the supposed effects different diets have on our bodies, ranging from performance to disease prevention. Our food plays a significant part in the maintenance of our health, in our bodies and in our relationships, and it's incredible what happens when you bring some awareness to these deeper parts of our lives.

There are all sorts of studies indicating something, and for every study saying one thing there is another stating the exact opposite. From eating for sports performance to eating for health to eating conscientiously toward our environment to sustainability of our livestock to the complete removal of any animal products, we humans have had a broad and varied diet throughout history. People bring up points about what we as humans have eaten for hundreds of years. Most of what we eat now has been tried and tested, and at least we know it doesn't kill us immediately, but our diet has ranged from an incredibly high-in-fibre diet, like the bushmen of some African tribes, or a diet almost completely devoid of vegetation, like that of the Inuit of the northern tundra, where there is little to no plant life in the frozen circle and the only vegetation might be that which is found in the stomach of some aquatic animals they catch. A professor of nutrition at Kansas State University lost twenty-seven pounds over ten weeks eating nothing but Hostess and Little Debbie snacks along with Doritos, sugar cereals, and Oreos. In traditional Chinese medicine they use "herbs" (parts of plants and animals) to heal the body, and they divide the herbs into two categories: superior and inferior. The inferior herbs include Ginseng or Gotu kola, which can only be taken for short periods due to their high potency. Prolonged exposure or use can lead to negative or undesirable side effects; for example, Siberian ginseng has been known to raise blood pressure and cause insomnia, vomiting, nosebleeds, and headaches, while the superior herbs are things like spinach, broccoli, chicken, celery, and such. These are fairly benign foods that can be consumed regularly and help to keep the body healthy and robust. This develops, heals, and sustains the body, but food crosses over into the other centres of operation as well.

Eating for the mind is in this category as well, as there are foods in certain cultures that are seen as teacher plants, that when eaten pass on information or help process and work through things from our past or present moments. There are foods for the mind, and we can see that food plays a part in how we think, not just how we perform, such as whenever we experience being hangry from having gone too long without food. Of course, the third operating-centre relationship is tremendously connected with food, since the earliest of times we have gathered, socialized and celebrated around eating.

Tension – Throughout life we will accumulate tension, and this can lead to pain and restriction in our bodies. Tension is an interesting thing inside of us, as with all the technology of the modern day we can see our bones with X-rays. With MRIs or CT scans we can observe our organs, and even our blood vessels and brain, and with ultrasound we can see if we have torn a muscle, but what we can't see with any of our diagnostic instruments is tension in a muscle, and yet we can see and feel it with our own eyes and hands. Tension is what produces the majority of discomfort we feel in our joints, but not all of it. Sometimes it's arthritis, sometimes it's related to the nerves. There can be many different causes for the pain and discomfort we feel, as pain is something that is poorly understood and yet still seems to be quite a subjective experience. It is difficult to rate pain aside from a personal interpretation, and the causes can reach even beyond the physical into psychosomatic roots.

So there can be many causes, but often a good portion of the discomfort and restriction we experience is due to tension where it can be addressed by bringing our awareness to it and trying to let it go, which is more difficult than it sounds. There are a variety of methods that we as human beings as a whole have found over the ages that seems to work. As it seems to be a good practice to bring awareness and variation to our nutrition and sleep, it would be useful to extend the idea of including a practice of awareness and variation for regularly taking care of and addressing the tension we incur inside ourselves through our lives. It is important to not only learn how to produce high levels of tension, but to learn how to let it go as well. We fight to hold on and we fight to let go, and it seems one way to let go of the tension is to first become aware of it, and once we become aware of it we can begin to figure out how to let it go.

Reflecting the Pyramid

As we apply a regular practice to exposing and challenging our bodies, we see that we begin to be able to make physical changes to the world, and that in turn creates physical changes in us. In this we bring the same focus to the mind. Our mind fills in the metaphysical. This is where it is full of ideas, and—much like the physical, where we can find ourselves stuck in cycles of repetition—as we change things our patterns change, so we get caught within thoughts constantly looping back to an old thought or experience from a traumatic moment in our life. Or we create negative self-talk, where we get caught in all the same trappings as the body but in a different way.

Great, so we can change the body, now how do we change the mind? How do we wake tomorrow and see things differently. Similar to the way we change the body, we can do it through exposure to new, different, and deeper ideas. We can dabble in interpretations and perspectives of our "existence".

Let's look back at Book 1, where the importance of inclusion of polarity was expressed in regard to the states of consciousness that we exhibit from a patriarchal perspective, valuing waking consciousness or sobriety. We don't want to operate a heavy machine while under the influence of anything, and yet there was also an acknowledgement from the matriarchal perspective of the many different altered states of consciousness that we are able to explore, as in the past we have made major decisions based on dreams, visions, and hallucinations. When we are in a sober and wakeful state, it can be difficult to just decide to see things differently, and regularly throughout history we have used altered states to induce a change in how we see and interpret existence. These practices spanned meditation, drumming, dancing, sensory overstimulation, sensory deprivation, sleep deprivation, fasting, and the widespread use of entheogens.

All of these help to break pattern of old, to release the hypnotic grip of the everyday trance. When we do something different, it separates the days, breaks patterns of old, and allows us to see a different world, to experience ourselves outside ourselves and inside ourselves as a bear, a raven, a tree, or a rock. As our paradigms change, we begin to be able to do more with our world than any one perspective alone could ever provide. As we shift into a different perspective we can see old patterns, and this can often allow us to become aware of these things we are doing in our lives, and we can start to make conscientious choices in dropping patterns that no longer serve us. It can help us see new patterns that couldn't be seen before. As American self-help author Wayne Dyer once said, "If you change the way you look at things, the things you look at change."

By far the most profound experiences seem to be derived from entheogens a.k.a teacher plants or psychedelics. This is currently still a relatively taboo subject, but it is gaining more momentum in the mainstream media as the research start to surface from universities such as Johns Hopkins and the University of Toronto to Harvard and Yale, to name a few, begin publishing their findings and seeing use for these substances in treating a number of mental health issues, from anxiety and depression to addressing trauma and cluster headaches effectively, with many more concerns such as Obsessive Compulsive Disorder and stuttering are being addressed anecdotally as claimed by American mycologist, Paul Stamets. There has been some research that suggests psychedelics can heighten the natural ability to form new associations and develop new behaviours (psymposia.com). There seems to be increased neural connectivity across many different regions of the brain, and even neurogenesis (the production of new neurons) has been observed from the use of psilocybin. There is a cessation of certain habitual thought patterns as well as the formation of new ones.

On an even more poignant note, the recent book by Michael Pollan titled *How to Change Your Mind* speaks of both his personal anecdotal experiences as well as what the leading sciences are showing us about what these substances do once inside our bodies and minds. From the applications, we are seeing treatment from end-of-life anxiety for cancer patients to depression and trauma. These substances seem to change the way we look at and perceive the things in our lives. Beyond the therapeutic applications, which are gaining more legitimacy as the research continues to come out, it is also being used for the purpose of disruption and challenge to shake up and stir the proverbial pot of the mind, as all too regularly people report being flooded with thoughts and imagery, ideas, and experiences that leave them wondering, *What was that?* As we try to grapple with the inconceivable, we stretch the limits of our minds and begin to open up to new possibilities.

In these types of practices there is a distinct element of uncertainty that we engage with that stirs the pot of the mind, bringing to the surface unforeseeable things. This keeps the pot good, so to speak, where there is a stimulation that aids in a rejuvenation that seems to help keep the mind spryer and more flexible, adaptable, and healthy. These experiences offer us an opportunity to experience our world differently, to experience ourselves differently, and in that there is the potential for new perspectives to be gleaned, thus broadening our vision so that we are able to see more possibility, and in that more freedom.

We are starting to put together the idea that our experiences shape our thoughts and that our thoughts shape our experiences. If we change our thoughts, we can change our experiences, and if we change our experiences, we can change our thoughts. So when it comes to Saturday night and we choose to do the typical thing we do every Saturday night, we tend to form the same experiences, and in that we habituate the same thoughts. Suddenly, we wonder how it's been seven years and still doing the same thing and living in the same rut. If we are wanting to change our minds, we must be willing to change our experiences in light of changing the way we think of our experiences.

With our minds often being the worst prison we could find ourselves in, it can be useful to break free of the walls we have built around us. Few things are set in stone, and when the mind can become our very own personal prison it is important to expose ourselves to new worlds of possibilities, and in that we see the possibility of reinterpreting our past to reengage with our present moment, and the possibility of rewriting our future.

With more and more research supporting the use of psychedelics (at least with mushrooms), they are currently being explored as tools to assist in problem solving, creative design, and writing in places like Silicon Valley, and assisting with performance enhancement which is being anecdotally reported by athletes in the WWE (World Wrestling Entertainment).. There is evidence of their use for hunting in certain tribes, and possibly by Viking berserkers before heading into battle. These substances have even been reported to be one of the few examples that could be linked to a true aphrodisiac. Currently these substances are being investigated for their possible use in treating addiction.

This is not to say that entheogens are the only way, as the primary goal is to disrupt thoughts and break patterns, and this can be done from fasting, going to sweat lodges, sensory deprivation, sensory overload, sleep deprivation, chanting, drumming, dancing, breathwork, meditation, fire walking, ice baths, body suspension—all things we don't do on a regular basis, and that's partly the point: engaging in these acts takes you out of your usual routine of life and breaks patterns, but these experiences provide a stretching of the senses, the mind, and ultimately ourselves.

We want to expose ourselves to things that challenge us in ways being a couch potato, wastefully lounging and binge watching television series don't do. It is for the sake of the strange and the weird that we partake in the obscene and bizarre, as we seem to understand more of the world and ourselves not when we look at what is consistent or normal but when things are different. Through this we gain a deeper and often more fascinating understanding. How often do we leave ourselves questioning, wondering, *What the fuck was that?* to instill a sense of wonder into ourselves. Like artwork that leaves you with more questions than answers, great experiences often leave us with few words when describing those experiences especially because they do not regularly exist in the mundane. Do weird things for the sake of keeping you from fading into the background and becoming part of the furniture.

So, what do you want to do this Saturday night?

Expanding the Sphere

Since we have been seeing how we might go about developing our bodies and opening our minds, we are going to see how we might go about expanding the heart. We have seen previously that to go about these processes we have stepped out of the conventional box of the body and the mind, but by exploring that through difficult experiences, we grow and become someone more than we were. As we shift our gaze inward to the heart, our practice goes outward into the world. You do not attain enlightenment sitting on the top of a mountain as Ram Dass once said "if you think you're enlightened, spend a week with your family", and it isn't necessarily found in the thick of things either as expressed in the value of venturing up into the mountain away from the masses below in the valley in Friedrich Nietzche's work Thus Spake Zarathustra: a book for all and none, but much like thus spake zarathustra it lies in the journeying between.

In the book *Sex at Dawn* by Christopher Ryan and Cacilda Jethá, the authors question the standard narrative of our human sexuality, which is men want to spread their seed and women want to find a provider and a protector. But when reviewing our history anthropologically, it seems that this scenario of man and woman never happened.

Back in hunter-gatherer times, you would never really see a single male and a single female running around in the woods.

We existed in and we co-habited as a wide and diverse support group. Even when we go back further into nature, monogamy seems less prevalent than previously believed. When citing monogamy in nature, birds are often pointed to for their noble ways, and people say, well, we see it in nature, humans must be monogamous by nature too. Since genetic testing has become considerably cheaper and much more readily available in the field, researchers have found that the majority of these birds partner for life, but when one is away the other will play. They saw this in the DNA matching of the chicks to the parents. When we bring the scope of nature to even our closest relatives, the chimpanzees and the bonobos, we see that neither of these species practice monogamy.

There is a river in the Congo. On the north side lives families of chimpanzees and on the south bonobos. Chimpanzees are patriarchal; they control the group through violence, aggression, and intimidation. The females are sexually active for 5 percent of their adult life, often having to separate themselves and leave the safety of the group during pregnancy and the early period of child rearing, as there is high level of infanticide which occurs in the group. The alpha male often has control of the females and will use them to gain favour within the group, allowing desired males access to females in return for collaboration.

On the other side of that river, the bonobos are matriarchal and control the group through sex. The females are sexually active for 55 percent of their adult life. Sexual favours abound, practices range from all types of acts on the spectrum without differentiating gender specific intimacies. It's used to calm social tensions and to re-enforce social bonds. Conflicts are resolved with hand jobs and orgasms. The groups are larger with no issues of infanticide since all kids are raised by the group.

Patriarchy seems to fragment the sisterhood and pit women against each other. Monogamy was a patriarchal construct designed to commodify women, like livestock, and it sought to control women's sexuality and ensure that the children they were going to provide for were indeed their own.

In Daniel Bergner's book *What Do Women Want? Adventures in the Science of Female Desire*, the author asks us to reconsider our long-held ideas of women's sexuality. Bergner draws from a number of scientific studies that ultimately ask us to question whether monogamy is best suited for women or not, with much of the findings directing us to look more at the latter than the former. He gives examples, such as one study from Australia that was investigating the women of the country who were postmenopausal due to their husbands complaining of a loss of libido, and a prevalent lack of the wives wanting to have sex with their husbands. After a lengthy investigation which looked at many factors that ran from diet to contaminants in the air, soil, and water to location of birth, to name but a few, they concluded that the only thing that seemed to act as an indicator was the duration of the relationship. The longer the relationship went on, the less interested the woman seemed to want sexual intimacy.

What was even more interesting was over the course of this study some of the women ended their relationship and started a new one, and wouldn't you know it? Her libido was right back to where it was. Studies using a device called a plethysmograph, which measures displacement of volume in an organ allowing for biometric readings to be observed, and it showed how prevalent desire is for women's arousal. It didn't matter what form of arousal was displayed; interestingly enough watching two bonobos going at it elicited a greater response in the genitals of the women watching than a video of a chiseled, naked man walking down a beach skipping a stone.

In her book *Mating in Captivity*, Esther Perel highlights two dominant and seemingly diametric forces that attract us in our relationships. We are drawn toward stability, predictability, and reliability, as these are valuable qualities to find when wanting to build a future that involves buying a house, starting a business, raising children, or whatever it is that we are pursuing. On the other hand, we are also drawn towards qualities of novelty, adventure, and mystery since they drive transcendence and offer opportunity for change.

Stability is dependable, and it is very important to have in life, but it can also become stagnant and this is the downfall of being predictable. The same can be said for its opposite. Being adventurous, mysterious, unpredictable, and spontaneous, living on the edge, never knowing where you are going to sleep, or being in a constantly changing landscape can be wearing and stressful, and so it seems there is something important to be said for both. Back to the idea of the coin, when we are able to find the space between the two, we are able to dance in ways neither side can do alone. There has always been tension between the individual and the group, between maintaining a sense of identity and being part of something more. Within intimate relationships, there is a balance between the *me* and the *us*. As Esther points out, "Love is to have and desire is to want," and within the very nature of coming upon something that is mysterious and unknown we want to spend more time getting to know the mystery, but the mystery fades and the closeness draws us in. The closeness can suffocate the flames of passion, as when Esther Perel shows in her observations that we are drawn to our partners when we see them as others do (someone else). For example, when our partner is on stage giving a speech or doing a performance for a crowd, it's independent of the relationship. It is when there is something more to discover that our curiosities are piqued.

If love is to have and desire is to want, then how do we want what we already have? We understand that we don't own our partners, and yet act as though we do. We expect the things we desire to stay fixed and remain unchanged without acknowledging the other's journey through time on this planet. British philosopher Alan Watts has been heard comparing it to learning how to swim: if you try desperately to hold on to the water you will sink and in all likelihood drown, but if you learn to relax and let go, you float, supported and carried by the very thing that was going to kill us. When we cling desperately to relationships, we smother, we become mundane and we often stop each other from living. We become fearful that the other will meet someone else and leave, so we cling to each other desperately, lovingly, and stagnantly.

We come alive the most when we don't know what to expect next. We can attend a theatre production of *I Love You, You're Perfect, Now Change* twenty times. There are potential obstacles and changes that can make it quite different all twenty times where accidents can occur, line are being forgotten, potential mechanical failures happen, actors who have fallen ill or have lost their voice completely and the list goes on. Each night is a once-in-a-lifetime performance, as it will be impossible to recreate exactly the same from one night to the next. A movie is highly refined and polished, with detailed angles and lighting with the best actors and the best makeup and the best take of a hundred, and all put together to make it magnificent but the first watch and the twentieth will all be exactly the same. But it's important to see that they both have their merits.

Marriage has a 50 percent divorce rate, but the remaining 50 percent who are still together does not speak of the people who are absolutely miserable and too scared end the relationship or are having affairs.

When looking across time and culture on this planet, we can see infidelity everywhere. No one has figured out how to evade the wandering eyes; no religion, no government, no degree of punishment has been able to prevent the curiosity which seems to come so natural for us. The question is begging to be asked: if we are monogamous by nature, why are we having such a hard time being what we naturally are?

The origins of monogamy were basically born out of owning property and seeing women as property to be owned for their sexual reproductive qualities, so that men could ensure the child was theirs. For a very long time, marriage had been more of a business contract of family partnering to guarantee power or finances, or to arrange a union so the children can have children. The idea of marrying for love is a relatively new concept, and this is the first time we are able to freely choose both our sexual interests and our life partners. We are still working out the kinks, so to speak since we are finding not all great lovers make great partners and not all great partners make great lovers. Once again we are reminded that this is not an "either or" instead a "both and." This is not a presentation of the opposite, but, as the title implies, it is something more of an amalgamation of the two.

What we start to see within the practice of the heart is that there are all sorts of areas of censorship that insert and interject themselves into our lives, but most disheartening is when we do it in our deepest and most intimate relationships. It is easy to point to areas within our primary relationships where we may be more inclined to inform our friends than our partners of our fantasies, if anyone else at all, and when it comes to sex it seems to reach deep to the core of us and reveal something true that we want to deny. For example, quite often in relationships we don't inform our partner when someone else catches our eye, or interesting conversations with someone who piques our interest, stirring something within. We deny it to our partners and we deny it to ourselves, and before we know it we are avoiding and skirting on side notes that may point toward the initial thing we were hiding from our partner, and the chasm grows and we move farther apart, and it becomes less and less of us we can reveal. When we invert the practice, where everything is on the table and there is no judgement (to the best of our abilities—we're human), there is a gushing and a flood ensues where so much more of ourselves can be revealed, shared, exposed, and accepted. There is a tremendous weight within us and within our relationships, and as we step into the light and start being our authentic selves it lets go, and that means getting to the core of ourselves. One way that can be effective at achieving a deeper level of authenticity is through sex itself, even just talking about it.

Within that practice is the first of many more opportunities to continue to step forward and have difficult conversations, in which we start saying the truth and not just what we think the other wants to hear. There are many conversations that we as humanity have not yet had, and in that there is a pioneering of sorts in discovering a new path, an authentic path, not one that is following a script or routine. As we talked about earlier in the first book about development, these are the challenges of the heart. Just like exposing ourselves to new stimuli and learning how to cope and manage, those new exposures allow us to grow to new heights and be able to play with greater freedom and grace. These are not easy things, but exposing ourselves to their challenges offers us more freedom within our lives for the future.

These experiences we step into often leave us humbled and humiliated, largely due to our own egos, and as we learn to manage these things we begin to move out of ourselves and be more considerate of other people. We no longer displace our sense of self to "me and my partner," but rather we include our partner's partner. This is not to say that I have to have an intimate relationship with my partner's partner, but to extend the idea that if I like myself and believe that I am a great person and my partner sees that in me, and there is someone else that has drawn the attention of my partner's heart, then I would hope that my partner has more great people in their life like me (not exactly like me, but a great human being). And if I am a great human being, would I not want the people that I love to be with great people? Whether these experiences are humbling or humiliating, we have opportunities to work through our emotions. We buckle and our insecurities get exposed so that we can work on those areas that need our attention.

When we find those areas that we could focus on to develop ourselves, like giving ourselves a haircut: it can be difficult to get at the back when we can only see the front. So when we are able to look at different views, we get an understanding of different parts of ourselves and become more complete than we were yesterday.

The Allegory of the Two Best Friends.

In these opportunities to work through our emotions, we come to the allegory of the two best friends in elementary school. These two friends do everything together: they spend recess together, they spend after school together, they do sleepovers on the weekends—they are practically attached at the hip. Then one day one of the friends meets another friend and runs off and spends the rest of the day with them. Meanwhile, the other friend is standing there throwing a tantrum. As an adult, we don't go over to the kid who is bawling their eyes out over this whole change of things and say, "Hey Jimmy [or Tina], you're absolutely right in how you feel. You should go over there and demand your friend leaves their new friend and spends the rest of the day with you." Instead we might say something like, "Hey Tina [or Jimmy], it's all right that your friend has just met a new friend. In fact, it might be a good idea for you to meet some new friends too. Don't worry, you can play with your old friend tomorrow." Unfortunately, when we grow up and we call that relationship "love," we suddenly feel justified to revert back to child-like tendencies. As an adult we rarely have the same opportunities to work through some of these things in life, and we never learn the lessons. The question begs to be asked: how do you work on things like jealousy without ever encountering them?

Through all of this, what begins to happen is a space opens between people in long-term relationships, where the flames of passion have been smothered to the point of the couple being more like sexless roommates or, worse, siblings, to return and grow again. As we begin to create some space, we are afforded the chance to redefine and explore ourselves and to see that we can change, and in changing identify a new take on an old source. When we go back to our partners, we have changed, we are someone new, there is a new landscape to explore, as with when we see our partner with a new hair colour or wearing something unexpected or new and we become intrigued again.

One thing that has been observed time and time again is when we do open up and play with others in an open and honest and consensual way and go back to being with our partner, sex between them is supercharged. We see couples over and over repeating the same reply: when going back afterward the intimacy is on fire, more than any piece of negligée or toy could bring, as it seems the space provided allows for the flames of passion that Esther Perel speaks of to grow to ravishing proportions.

Applying the analogy of the disease of *mono* (of oneness, not mononucleosis meningitis), we can see in many different aspects of life that when we repeat the same thing over and over, good things come at first, but if pursued too much those things that gave us a boom become our bust. When we look into movement, we can see that repeating the same one can produce a repetitive strain or a muscular imbalance across a joint. In the same training program, you can have stagnation. Eating the same thing over and over leaves us depleted of other nutrients we would get from a diversity of foods. When we have repeated thoughts, they come to be considered obsessive thoughts, and those don't seem to be desirable. Within the gene pool, we can see with thoroughbred animals where there is an emphasis that is placed on certain features that are desirable, and to achieve those traits inbreeding is used. As the gene pool grows smaller and smaller, ever more "pure" diseases begin to show up, and again diversity seems to yield a deeper gene pool to draw from, producing greater variants of genes that allow for a more adaptable species. Within farming, the same crop grown over and over again in the same field will deplete the soil, hence the reason farmers employ crop-rotation methods. We can see over and over in many different areas of life that when we do something too much it becomes problematic. Why do we exclude our heart from this idea? We can see that it makes no sense to ask someone to pick one book to read for the rest of their life—that would almost be a crime. To ask someone to pick one movie for the rest of their lives, or to eat one dish, doesn't make sense, so why do we say that it makes sense with our hearts? Is it because of the difficulty of facing our emotional beasts and the learning curve it takes to approach this? But if we do, we start to soar to unimaginable heights, just as we are able to perform ever more impressive physical feats with our physically developed bodies. We will be able to demonstrate such feats with our emotionally developed heart as well, when we learn to develop it in the same way we develop the body.

In this whole practice, there is a journeying of sorts that brings us between venturing out into uncharted, unfamiliar territories, all the while returning home to find a sense of being grounded and stable that we sort of reference as a north star. There is an interaction between the tensions that arise as new triggers are stepped on, and there is newfound freedom in learning to relax into this discomfort. Much like tension in the body, we rarely find it on our own. When we engage in this type of practice, we tend to find all sorts of triggers that can help or hinder, depending on how it is approached. There is acknowledgment to preserving something within consistency that allows us to build and develop, but to also experience variation and change within an ever-changing world. We form patterns, but it is easy to get stuck within them, and these practices often help to highlight when we repeat our inauthenticity, and they help to introduce new patterns and disrupt the old, helping to stir the pot. It's not all play; there is serious and uncomfortable work that accompanies this practice, as it asks us to connect while being willing to let go.

Dutch extreme athlete Wim Hof, the famous Iceman, is still redefining (as of 2020) our scientific understanding of exposure to extremely cold temperatures. Through breath work and exposure, he advocates a slow and progressive non-forced exposure to achieve tolerance to cold temperatures previously thought unattainable, and this is where curiosity comes into play. This is not to say that there is some mandatory partner rotation or institutionally imposed exchange; again, these are extremes and ridiculous practices to implement. But we should have a degree of honesty and authenticity within ourselves and our conduct with each other so that we allow ourselves to explore, as often things that initially catch our interests quickly burn out and we start to refine our interests or begin to see our patterns. As we become more cognizant of our inner workings, we refine ourselves.

We see over and over in many different aspects of life that great things come when we step up to challenge adversity within our bodies and minds, so why not our hearts as well? There have been enough anecdotal stories of growth being stimulated from these challenging excursions, a cultivation of valued authentic behaviour, and a genuine care for our fellow human beings as well as ourselves through these experiences.

Conclusion

This isn't a blueprint of answers but rather paths to explore along this journey we call Life. In this journeying, we begin to stretch our boundaries and redefine our spaces and relocate our centre. When we have more experiences to draw upon, to navigate ourselves in this wild and crazy world, we are more grounded. In this there is no radical revision suggesting a heavy swing to the other side, or that we are against order or for chaos or any of that. This is more in line with what Buddha was referencing with the middle path, where we are not suggesting one or the other but rather something in between, and what makes that in-betweenness so difficult is that it's constantly changing and shifting, like the shape of a bubble or a flame, where its shape is in constant flux and the surface swirls like a maelstrom on a planet seen from above. With this bubble/flame there is a consistent shape, and yet that shape constantly changes from moment to moment, never staying the same, and yet is always a bubble or a flame. In this it will be different for everyone at different times, and nothing stays the same. By journeying between concepts and ideas, we find a continuous potential for growth and development. As we let go of any one thing, we begin to see we exist between the spaces of things and identities, and in seeing that we are able to let drop who we thought we were. We see we are able to pick up who we might want to become. This is merely to provide boundaries for us to explore the spaces between, and see that we occupy much more than any one stance ever could.

Book 3

The How

THE FIRST BOOK WAS HEAVILY philosophical, speaking of the *why* behind the idea of journeying between two polarized points in many different ways, and that the balance we seek is more akin to the spin of a coin or the balance of a bicycle: it's in motion, a dynamic balance rather than static. In the second book we began to speak more specifically about what we are talking about and what that might look like. Now, finally, we are at the third book, where we will be discussing how do we go about the things we were suggesting in the second book.

This is to merely act as an example of how one might go about plotting a course after having read the first two books. By no means is this meant to be something set in stone, but hopefully something more progressive and evolutionary, to be referred to as things go on and grow in complexity. We begin to see the need to grow into something else rather than what was necessary. This is all to simply suggest one way of many ways, as this is a lifelong journey of development that moves progressively from yin to yang and back again. It is in the exchange between the two that we become static and still, much like the spin of a hubcap or the blades of a helicopter: at a certain speed the spin of the wheels or the rotation of the blades begin to look still while in motion.

At the end of the day these are only ideas to work with as we explore reality, as what speaks to each of us may be different. These very same principles can be applied across the board as to what we would like to expose ourselves to.

We are looking to reorganize how we act, think, and relate, and in changing those things we will be looking at breaking patterns. In acknowledging that our past experiences, environments, thoughts, and relationships have influenced us greatly in how we currently act, think, and feel, we have the potential to free ourselves from the patterns that have kept us so habitually locked in to a destiny that we don't want and yet continually choose to put ourselves in. In knowing that our past has shaped and formed who we are and how we act, the onus is on us to realize that what we do now will become the past that shapes us in the future, and in becoming cognizant of that fact we can willingly choose to become who we are.

We can see that, physically speaking, our current body is composed of all our past events to varying degrees leading up to this moment, from our physique to our physical health to the way we move. We can see that our past and all the things that happened to us or didn't happen to us have accrued in our bodies, and this shows us that what we do now will produce our body in the future, and that we can take the lead of our own growth and choose to develop and grow to become more capable than we were yesterday.

We certainly see that our thoughts affect how we see and interact with the world at large. If we continue to tell ourselves how worthless or pathetic we are, or how much no one wants or cares for us, or how much the world is against us, it can certainly paint the world in some fairly unpleasant colours. When we go back and examine where these thoughts are playing like a broken record, we see that something from our past has set us in motion to think this way and see the world as we do today. As much as this can seem frustrating or daunting, we can see that what we think and experience today will shape how we think of the world and ourselves in the future giving us a chance to create a version of ourselves that we would like tomorrow.

The parallels of the two above ideas for the body and the mind hold true for the heart as well. There have been enough tropes in stories to become aware of the idea that we often find ourselves in a relationship that was just like the last one, as it seems we frequently pick relationships largely based on past experiences that have set us up in motion to repeat, whether it's pursuing someone like our parents or that we are trapped in a cycle of abusive relationships. Our relationships from the past play a crucial role in our current relationships, and if our previous relationships affect and form our decisions and actions in our current relationships, then we know that our current relationships will affect the decisions and actions of our relationships in the future.

Knowing that our past in many ways affects and influences us today, and considering we want to change how we act, think, and feel, then let's not repeat the same mistakes we have made in the past. That is not to say we will pick the best answers moving forward, because we don't know the answers, especially as our present world changes at an exponential rate. We are faced with new situations where the old answers no longer suffice, and yet the idea here is not to throw the baby out with the bath water either. Stepping forward into the future of uncertainty requires a certain degree of pliability, spontaneity, and thinking on your feet, and those are qualities that are difficult to teach. One way to go about this is through exposure, through diverse experiences. It offers us a reservoir to draw from, and the accumulation of perspectives gives us a multitude of ideas to play around with in our universe. Through our engagement with various forms and types of relationships, we understand more about ourselves.

As you continue reading, you'll find suggestions on how to explore and venture down this path of self-development. This journey is extremely personal and subjective, what may appeal or pique the interests of one person may not carry over to another, and none of these suggestions are to be seen as the answer to everything. So with your curiosity and courage, the aim of this book is to encourage you, the active reader, to journey and explore in many ways unique to you. There isn't a person out there who has all the answers but we can come together as a group and offer a collective blueprint of trials, experiences, and results of the life that we want for ourselves and each other.

The Cube

In this section we are going to discuss a variety of tools, techniques, and concepts that we can use to explore and develop our physical bodies. The website www.geoffhunnef.com will offer more information and explanations to this section.

1. Internal movement
Physical meditations, reflective explorations of biomechanical movements. This is much more internal, both in the mind and the body, requiring sensitivity to become aware of and feel the subtle differences in regard to the internal alignment. Some examples of these would be D.K. Yoo's Cham Jang Gong technique, the Feldenkrais Method, or the Alexander Technique.

2. External movement
These are the large gross movements that are the typical ones we see in sports, when we move a limb, skip a stone, drink coffee from a cup, or massage someone. Examples would be running, jumping, wrestling, bench pressing, climbing, etc.

3. Open-chain movements
These would be anything that involves moving our limbs instead of our torso. Examples would be pressing or pulling

motions using dumbbells, barbells, kettle bells, cables, leg presses, lat pulldowns, the use of clubs or maces, or throwing an object. This include all variations of bench presses, shoulder presses, flys, raises, bent rows, leg presses, leg curls, leg extensions, bicep curls, and triceps extensions using an external load and moving the limbs while the torso remains stationary. Ie: Moving things around you.

4. Closed-chain movements

These would be anything that is moving the torso around the limbs. These include all variations and permutations of deadlifts, squats, push-ups, dips, handstand presses, pull-ups, body rows, natural leg curls and extensions, levers, and planches. Ie:Moving you around things

5. Alive movements

An alive movement is continuous and in one direction, never reversing and returning the way it came. The tools that are most easily used for this type of work are clubs and maces. These tools are not so common in the West, yet clubs and mace training are probably two of the oldest forms of training with an external load we can find historically, as these replicated the use of weapons like swords or clubs to help develop combative strength and mobility.

These can be swung in a single line, but where these tools seem to separate from conventional barbell or dumbbell technique is that you can continue the movement in a circle, always moving in the same directions, or in a figure 8. These tools can help to develop better strength and mobility in the shoulders. As you can get clubs weighing up to 40 lbs, these movements also help to develop the idea of flow, where there is continuous seamless transitionary movement allowing for a continuous and changing movement.

6. Dead movements

"Dead" has a negative connotation, but this is to simply indicate that the movement has come to an end point and is to return the way it came, in reverse. These movements are like deadlifts, curls, push-ups, kettle-bell swings, triceps extensions, bench presses, pull-ups . . . and the list goes on. These are almost all other conventional lifts.

7. Intensity

"Intensity" is dealing with any of the movements that we are already able to perform where we increase the intensity, which translates as load within the context of strength and conditioning. So, deadlifts, bench presses, curls, kettle-bell swings, loaded push-ups, dips, etc. These tend to be the usual way most people think about developing ourselves physically.

8. Complexity

"Complexity" is where we are progressing our training to be able to perform a movement that we were previously unable to execute. Examples would be moving from a push-up to a pseudo-planchet push-up to a bent planchet hold to full planchet push ups, where you perform a push up while holding your feet up suspended in the air supported by nothing; parallel bar dips to a single bar dip to a Korean bar dip to rings dip; a hanging leg lift to a kip on a bar to a front leaver. These are where we are unable to do a movement on a first attempt, but with time and dedication and proper development we are able to perform a movement that we couldn't imagine executing when we first attempted it.

9. High tension

These are exercises that teach us to fill the body with tension from tip to toe, allowing for us to perform some incredible feats. Exercises that require full-body tension are mostly any of the gymnastic movements or deadlifts. When the stress on the body exceeds a certain level, we have a full and recruited body that comes to life. This is induced by exposing ourselves to high intensity via load or complexity.

10. Low tension

This is the opposite of the above. Instead of using every fibre in our bodies to connect and tie in, trying to find ways our toes can be used to help curl up that weight in our arms, we are trying to use just the muscles that are necessary to complete the movement, making for subtle and energy-efficient movements. This is seen in some training systems like Systema, where there is a significant emphasis on relaxation and letting drop the unneeded tension.

There is a time for high and a time for low, and it seems to be a good idea for us to learn when, where, and why we would want to have access to one or the other, so it looks to be a good idea to explore and hold both in mind.

11. Structured

Structured movement is where we have structure to what we are learning, like a set routine, a set curriculum. This could be seen in *katas* in martial arts and forms in gymnastics, but this also goes into the way it is taught as well as where there is an expectation of having certain criteria acquired before the next step. This can be slower and more tedious, but it can help to detail out and keep a consistency within what is being taught and how it is being understood. This is most forms of learning where there is something given by the instructor, and the student replicates it back.

12. Unstructured

"Unstructured" is where the learning is more in the abstract and left more to the student or specific guidance from the instructor. Examples of these could be seen in Systema or breakdancing on the streets.

As it has been said before, we can move from form to formlessness or from formlessness to form, but it is important to keep in mind that, much like standing upright, it is how we engage in the world and mainly interact with it. When we go upside down, we start to gain from perceiving the same thing inverted. When we flip the script, as much as it's different, it's the same, and as much as it's the same, it is different. Both hold value in the spaces in between.

13. Solo work

"Solo work" is anything that we practice or explore by ourselves. Working out in the conventional sense in a gym can be solo work, as when we lift a weight. Even with a spotter it's not seen entirely as a team effort, but this too is a quality to observe. Just doing a solo workout by ourselves or with a partner changes the dynamics, and both show values to be aware of and include. Solo work is anything that does not require the involvement of another person, regularly pertaining to things like shadow boxing, resistance training, swimming, katas, hitting pads, running—generally anything that won't change in the moment.

14. Partnered work

This is anything that involves a partner: sparring, dancing, any team sports, and such. As soon as you train with another person, the workout changes for the better, and sometimes for the worse, but all of it adds more experiences to draw from and extends into ever more abstract ideas, such as the example of being paired with a partner you don't enjoy working with. This may not help you in the moment of developing your lift or executing a movement, but instead it challenges you to learn how to navigate unpleasant people, or how to become a better teacher. The lessons run so much deeper than just the physical ones if we are open to them.

15. Competitive

Within partnered work we can engage with others, either competitively or cooperatively. Competitive engagement can help push us to newfound limits, as the competitive edge is the evolutionary drive in the arms race, so to speak.

16. Cooperative
This is where there is an understanding between the people involved that they are intentionally trying to help each other improve and become better, as each person is attentive to the level at which the other is working, as the learning is curved toward each person's skill set.

17. Abstract hindrances
This is to allow a study of movement, not from giving something to look at or engage with, but rather by taking tools away. We become more open to new ways of things when we can no longer fall back on our conventional ways of doing them. If we spend the day with one arm tied behind our back or with one leg in a locked position, we become more aware of things that we wouldn't normally have picked up, as these help us tap into the nuances and subtleties of movement and help us to open our mind to new possibilities in our kinetic abilities.

Here is a list of tools we can incorporate into our training, and again this is by no means an exhaustive list, but more things to be aware of and include in the exploration of movement with our bodies.

Tools
- Barbells, dumbbells, kettle bells, club bells, maces
- Bulgarian bags, parallettes, parallel bars, horizontal bars, vertical bars, ropes
- Rings, people, pravilo, silks, hoops, chairs, sticks

Styles
- Gymnastics, calisthenics, pole fitness, hand balancing, circus, yoga, Pilates,
- Weightlifting, power lifting, strong man, strength and conditioning, body building, CrossFit
- Acroyoga, low acrobatics, acrobatics, parkour

Cardio
- Running, skipping, cycling, rowing, swimming, hills/stairs
- Trampoline, walking

Combative
- Systema, Brazilian jiu-jitsu, Silat, Shastar Vidya, capoeira, wrestling
- Muy Thai, judo, tai chi chen, aikido, boxing, fencing, Historical European martial arts

Dance
- Hip hop, ballet, breakdancing, contemporary, jazz, butoh, salsa
- Merengue, line dancing, tap dancing, lion dancing

Leisure
- Rock climbing, kayaking, hiking, canoeing, swimming, skating
- Skiing, biking

Abstract hindrance
- Restrict an arm, restrict a leg, restrict a direction, restrict vision
- Work with disadvantages

Body work
It is important that we also take care of our bodies, with all the activity that we do in our lives and the stresses that accumulate from time to time. Take the time to give some care and nurture to the thing that does so much for us our bodies.

- Traditional Chinese medicine, ayurvedic medicine, Slavic medicine, chiropractic medicine
- Qigong, massage, breath work, meditation, sauna, ice baths

Types of Eating
- Paleo, vegan, carnivorous, pescatarian, fasting, feasting
- Food for function, food for health (prevents disease, infection, parasites), spiritual food, conscientious moral and ethical eating

Sleep
Normal uninterrupted sleep, polyphasic sleep, sleep Deprivation, naps

These are to bring awareness and a sense of direction when we are left treading water and don't know where to go next. If you have a sense of where to go, then by all means follow your nose. The advice here is to engage and explore and to keep on exploring when one thing grows tired or we feel we can't go on any further in that particular field due to injury, age, or lack of ability, then set it down and pick something else up and keep expanding, keep being the new kid. There is so much to discover in the world and within ourselves that unless we want to stop, there is no objective end goal in mind. There is to be no grasping, only engaging and exposing. The only thing we try is to expose ourselves to new and different things, not to desperately achieve the handstand or to deadlift 405 lbs or the 225 lbs clean and press overhead, because often in reaching and grasping for these things we think we need or want, they do not bring us any more happiness or joy as our gaze settles upon the next feat. It never ends. There is no more happiness in squatting 495 lbs for the first time compared to squatting 225 lbs for the first time, but there is happiness in health and sadness in sickness, so move and explore and be happy with your discoveries along the way.

The Pyramid

We have been able to see how when we change our physical environment, such as taking a skill set like surfing from a surfboard on water to the snowy alps to snowboard or a park to skateboard. As we change the environment while keeping the primary movement the same, new things become revealed. As we see things and experience things differently, our bodies adapt and change to our environment. The same can be said for the mind as well. When we expose ourselves to different environments and experiences, they affect the way we think and perceive the world and ourselves in it. Knowing that our environment and the experiences we have in those spaces have influences, we can start to choose and create the types of experiences we want to have in them. This isn't to say we should go and do a Star Wars–themed birthday party at a Chuck E. Cheese, though we could, but we are really speaking of deeper and stranger things. This isn't just to shake things up and look at things differently, but also to see what lurks in the shadows of ourselves, as the subconscious is a part of ourselves we rarely learn how to engage with.

We tend to think we operate on a basis of logic and rational thinking, though much of our decision making is handled by the subconscious, and it is an irrational mind. How often do we say one thing and then do another? "I'm going to quit today," we say, and fast forward six weeks later and we are back doing the same routine. Our subconscious speaks more through metaphors, symbols, and senses than words alone, so how do we engage with this part of ourselves? Through meditation and dreams, art, and plants, we begin to pierce through the veil and see what's behind the curtain. There are many ways, but here we will cover only a few, and the reasons we might partake in some of these practices.

1. Breath work

We begin to see how much of our mind is connected to breath when we speed our breathing up or slow it down. We see how many functions in the body change when we change our breathing, and as we change our physiology we also begin to change our psychology, as the two are intimately connected. At times it can seem as though our body and our mind are divided when our bodies do things we wish they wouldn't. The crossroads where body and mind meet is our breath. It's crucial from the time our mothers were breathing for us when we were in the womb to the moment we take our first breath on our own to the time we breathe out our last. Our breath is a constant, and it is something we can use and manipulate.

There are all sorts of breathing exercises that span the globe, from performance enhancement like Russian hyper-breathing, to free-diving breathing exercises, to meditative breathing like holotropic breathwork and alternate-nostril breathing (nadi shodhan pranayama).

There are many different ways to breathe, and when we bring our awareness to our regular and consistent breathing and play around with it, we discover new and profound aspects of ourselves. If we start to breathe rapidly, we amp up our nervous system and saturate our blood with oxygen, getting everything ready for action. Our heart starts to pump harder as if we were running, and the blood circulates faster. It increases our metabolism and stimulates the mind. When we slow our breath down, it calms all those same functions and quiets the mind and depresses the nervous system instead of exciting it, all through breath. When we choose to breathe, our consciousness indicates cues to the body and stimulates or depresses certain functions. With the inversion of the same idea, we can see how when certain things happen to our body it causes our breathing to change, and as our breathing changes so does our psyche. If we perceive a threat to ourselves, to our body or otherwise, and we feel like things may break into a fight, our muscles tense up, hormones surge, and our breathing changes as we begin to enter our fight or flight mode, and often the state of mind that we are beginning to enter into is panic. So you can see how this flows in both directions. We can have things happen to our body that affects our mind and we can do things in our mind to affect our body, and our breath is the most immediate and simple thing for us to engage with.

Here are some examples of breathing exercises, both solo and partnered, curtesy of Vladimir Vasiliev, head instructor at Systema's Toronto headquarters.

1. Solo work

Begin walking continuously. While walking, start taking one breath in for a step and one breath out for a step. Then take two steps per in-breath and two steps per out-breath. Then three steps per one in-breath and three steps per one out-breath. Continue this pattern, working up to twenty steps per in-breath and twenty steps per out-breath, as this helps us to stretch out our lungs and teaches us to ration our breath and how to manage it, always paying attention to whatever comes up physically and psychologically.

2. Partnered work

Partner A lies on the floor face up while partner B kneels down at the side of partner A, facing them. Partner A takes a deep breath and pushes all their air out until there is no air in the lungs, and then holds their empty breath, all while partner B continues to wait until partner A can't hold their breath any longer. When partner A begins gasping for air, partner B starts hitting, slapping, choking, and trying to disrupt and challenge partner A's breathing, while partner A's job is to recover their breath and return to normal, paying little to no attention to partner B. Once partner A has recovered, switch. Again, observe any and all things that come up from the experience on both sides. Both partners have to observe internally, as well as observing and watching their partner.

3. Challenges to the form

These practices stretch the mind by stretching the body, through such things as hooked suspensions, like the sun-dance ceremonies of the indigenous plains people of

North America and other cultures around the world, to fire-walking ceremonies from various cultural practices ranging from New Zealand and Japan to India and Bulgaria. Ice baths are popular in Nordic traditions from Finland to Siberia, and are now becoming popularized by Wim Hof and his introduction of the Wim Hof Method, where he has been defying what science has confirmed for years: the body's ability to withstand the elements is far greater than we thought where it shows us the body is far more capable than we believed, and we can begin cracking open the mind to the understanding that maybe reality isn't quite what we thought it was.

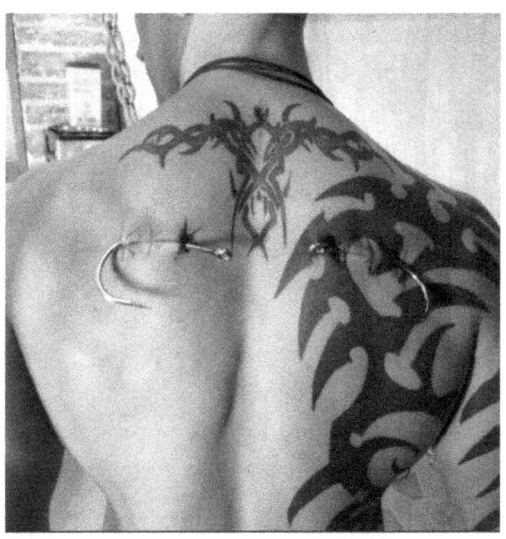

4. Entheogens

This is the widespread use of what some cultures call "teacher plants." The research coming out of Johns Hopkins University, among other contemporaries, is confirming that these things in one way or another have a profound effect on helping to heal the mind, allowing for insights to be seen that previously were not, to the discovery that they have neurogenic properties as well. These substances have been in use for long periods and in many different ways. These reasons have ranged from performance enhancement physically, intellectually, and creatively, as there have been reports of hunters using psilocybin (mushrooms) for hunting. Vikings report having berserkers who would consume a concoction containing Amanita muscaria, another entheogenic fungi. Hunters in South America would feed Psilocybe cubensis to their dogs to aid in the hunt, as their senses became heightened. Modern-day wrestlers in the WWE anecdotally report the use of micro-dosing mushrooms during their training for physical performance enhancement. Silicon Valley has been reporting the use of micro-dosing psychedelics for enhanced problem solving and creative design solutions, not to mention it's one of the hottest topics in mental wellness circles for helping with low energy and mild depression.

At moderate to higher doses beyond the micro-dose, we start to see that in regard to addressing depression, anxiety, PTSD, cluster headaches and possibly stuttering, according to rockstar mycologist Paul Stamets, as the research coming out is showing the use of the substances alongside guided therapy has had far greater effects at making a change for the patients than twenty years of conventional talk therapy and anti-depressant medication. In the more abstract still, it offers a reshuffling of sorts with perspectives. We can't help but look at things differently, as it distorts or removes the filters we keep so diligently up in our waking life that we never take the time to see what's behind the curtain. It has been a profound tool in helping to see the unpleasant things about ourselves that are so often skirted around in conversation with another. While in the grip of an introspective experience, it is difficult to look away from something that is being shown in the forefront of our minds.

Gabor Mate, a Hungarian-born Canadian physician and addiction expert, speaks of how our understanding of addiction was based on getting a rat addicted to cocaine-laced water and then putting it into a cage with cocaine-laced water and normal water and nothing else. Of course, the rat just did cocaine until it died, largely because it was a rat in a cage with nothing else to do. The same study was repeated in 2010 by Bruce K. Alexander, professor Emeritus, Simon Fraser University, where the scientist would establish an addictive behaviour to cocaine-laced water as well, but this time they would put the addicted rat into a rat park with lots of other rats (they are social creatures) and plants and objects to interact with, and it showed that the rats isolated in a cage with nothing else consumed much more of the drug-laced water than the other rats that were placed in the park.

Entheogens have been shown as a useful tool in treating addiction, but interestingly it doesn't seem to be a "take two and call me in the morning" sort of thing, as the usefulness of these substances have been linked to an experience on these fauna that is more than just a matter of taking a handful of fungi. The experience that seems to yield such positive results is known as the "mystical experience," described as "universal oneness," where the person reports feeling at one with the universe where boundaries dissolve, or as though everything is as its supposed to be. This is reported from other experiences too. It could be during a religious ceremony in prayer, it could be in meditation, but it seems to most reliably and consistently show while imbibing these substances.

This is not to say these are a panacea; it isn't that these things heal us, but they offer us insight into ourselves at times showing us a new perspective, a different angle to look at our past and seeing things differently may start to change the way we tell ourselves our story.

Even if it isn't necessarily for healing purposes, one can still benefit from an annual practice of venturing into our minds and seeing what lies below the surface.

The potential of the substances is to disrupt and break patterns of our minds away from how we see the world to how we see ourselves, to the language we use when no one else is around to hear what we say to ourselves behind closed doors.

These substances can be taken on the micro-dosing level to help with mood and energy or working out and training. There is a growing awareness both in the academic world as well as the public sphere of the use and benefits of these compounds for a plethora of applications, and the anecdotes continue to grow as the scientific committee begins to weigh in.

On moderate doses, we can experience it in both ways. We can keep it static and stationary where we sit and allow our minds to ruminate deeply into topics and ideas. The other way, we can venture out into the world on a spirit walk. Both ways can be done either alone of with a guide (someone who is very experienced with this). Spirit walks are often done at night, as during the day the light can be very illuminating, allowing our sharpened vision to see things in a sort of hyper-realistic way, where the world seems edged with a glimmer of magic. The world can seem very beautiful and inviting, but also very distracting, while at night when we walk into the darkness the shadows and lighting act as a proverbial Rorschach inkblot, allowing the inner machinations of the mind to be cast on the world around us. As we look out into the world, we begin to peer back into ourselves. The walks are often curated by someone beforehand who knows the path to walk and is able to offer guidance and security in troubling or difficult points along the journey. Venturing out and stepping into the unknown almost acts as re-enactment of what Joseph Campbell called "The Hero's Journey," often returning with pearls of wisdom after having faced our inner demons and confronted our shadows in the night.

Larger amounts go up to incredibly high degrees with things like psilocybin, where people like researcher Kilindi Iyi reach doses of up to thirty grams of dried mushrooms. These levels are reserved for the more experienced practitioners. It has been recommended at these levels that we venture into these parts alone, as it seems whenever we are in the presence of another, no matter how familiar or comfortable we are, a mask is worn. In this practice of looking to remove the layers, so to speak, of the masks we wear in society, we begin to see ourselves, and in this regard it seems these matters are best pursued alone.

In these undertakings we can come upon some difficult and challenging moments, such as when we encounter what Carl Gustav Jung called our "shadow." In dealing with shadow work, we must encounter our darker and less desirable qualities, as it is difficult for us to look at something we don't really want to see. We avoid the mirror, afraid to see the monster within, and yet far too often we are afraid to see all the scars and hideous markings, which aren't actually us but rather the breaks in the mirror that distorted our reflection. When we mend the mirror, we start to see the beauty that's both inside and out. It all starts with seeing the monster within and confronting the things we secretly think we are, coming face to face with the things we hate most about ourselves. This can be a difficult task for even the most skilled therapists, as you can bring a horse to water but you can't make them drink. Just because the therapist has pointed out an issue that could be worked on doesn't mean the person being helped sees what the therapist sees. When we go into our own minds and our shadow steps into the forefront and we see it with our mind's eye in all of its terrifying glory, we can't look away or close our eyes or pretend we didn't hear the question or divert the conversation.

In all this, what we are looking to accomplish is to disrupt and break the pattern of how we see things, and this begins the cracking of the mind's walls. What was once seen as an absolute, starts to show that maybe we don't have all the answers, maybe the world isn't what we thought it was, and perhaps we are not who we thought we were. With these questions starting to rise to the surface we start to look and investigate and become more curious about what's going on around us, since it no longer seems to be what we thought it was.

5. Mummification and pseudo death rites

Alan Watts said, "Everybody should do in their lifetime, sometime, two things. One is to consider death. To observe skulls and skeletons and to wonder what it will be like to go to sleep and never wake up—ever. That is a most gloomy thing to contemplate. It's like manure. Just as manure fertilizes the plants and so on, so the contemplation of death and the acceptance of death is very highly generative of crating life. You'll get wonderful things out of that. The other thing is to follow the possibility of the idea that you are totally selfish. That you don't have a good thing to be said for you at all. You are a complete and utter rascal."

Thinking about and reflecting on such matters is likened to manure, in that in itself it isn't pretty to look at nor pleasant-smelling, and on its own we don't want much to do with it, but damn it, this is the stuff that flowers grow from . . .

With that in mind, this area starts to deal with existential experiences that bring to light deep philosophical questions to reflect upon and to integrate into our daily lives. These would be acts of mummification, where someone is cast inside plaster of Paris, spending up to three hours inside a cast where they can't hear, move, and see, while reflecting upon the reality that one day we will die and everyone we know will die. Or go for a walk through a cemetery at midnight. This may seem somewhat macabre or dark, but much like the Stoics it is in these practices that we find inspiration to pick ourselves up rather than to be weighed down by heavy thoughts. In Dante Alighieri's poem *Divine Comedy*, Virgil, a guide for Dante's journey into hell and purgatory, said, "Death twitches my ear; 'live,' he says . . . 'I am coming.'" This is to remind us of the relentless pressing onwards of the march of time moving us ever closer to the moment we shuffle off this mortal coil, and in that we may be moved to act in bigger ways, to make larger splashes, to hold our loved ones closer and speak our hearts more authentically. Unfortunately, we wait too long to hear about the coming of our own death, knowledge which causes a sort of refocusing of our eyes onto the things that seem to truly matter to us. If we can become more cognizant of this fact, we might be so bold as to live as though one day we will die, and with that in mind speak, think, and act as though we are alive.

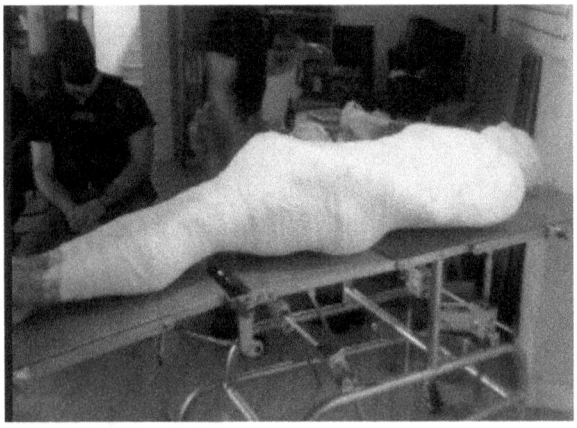

Just like the abstract hindrances in the physical operating system, there are exercises that yield some interesting observations for the mind as well. Instead of blocking a physical part of ourselves, we can borrow some suggestions from the likes of English occultist Aleister Crowley, where we create restriction and hindrances in our mind. For this the recommendation would be to spend a day or a week with the restriction or prohibition of using certain words, such as "the," "and," or "but," and see how in the avoidance we have to alter our thoughts and our speech to come up with new and creative ways to communicate. Another suggestion was to wear a marker of sorts, a ring or a bracelet, and when we move the marker from one hand to the other or from one finger to another, we invert our personality or our character. There are many ways this could be interpreted, and arguably each interpretation of how we go about inverting will yield new and unforeseen gems or pearls of wisdom for us to observe and incorporate as we see fit. Again, we can see from the disruption of patterns new things come about and allow us not to just discover new things but to see old things in new ways.

The Sphere

We have seen how our bodies change to meet the demands that we expose them to, and that by adversity, difficulty, dedication, and intention we can change ourselves physically. If we are able to apply the same strategy to our mind, we begin to see that, to paraphrase Wayne Dyer, when we change the way we look at things, the things we look at begin to change, and if we have been able to change our bodies—and by that, change our minds—we begin to see that perhaps we can change our hearts too. In changing our hearts, we begin to change our relationships, and this means learning to step forward into vulnerability, revealing our inner selves.

One of the things that seems to come up more and more is this aspect of loneliness, a sense of separation that seems to be running through North American civilization. It is odd that people can be in a metropolis surrounded by millions of people and feel so alone, with a sense of isolation so great that the option of committing suicide seems more logical than to continue marching onward, following in line, and when people do rise up and step out of line, society wonders why, and the answer seems obvious. Why get out of line? Because this line is marching toward our death. We sit in our homes day after day, week after week, passing the time by watching actors on a screen in front of sets made in Hollywood warehouse basements. The series writers have gotten the formula down to a T, and can set the hook deep with such shows as *Game of Thrones* or *Breaking Bad*. We get sucked in and commit to binge-watch series with something like seventy-three episodes, with the average run time per episode of an hour—that's seventy-three hours. The reality of this is highlighted by the question, "How was episode thirty-five?" Not many people would be able to recollect what happened in that specific one, let alone having it make a significant and positive effect on their lives. We spend too much time in front of screens and not interacting with people. This isn't an attack on television or entertainment, it's just to say that with all of the great programming that's going on nowadays, the most influential or significant and meaningful moments in our lives will not come from being in front of a screen. If I want a life of meaning, then it certainly means getting out and away from the screen that we spend so much time with. We live in a time where screens are stealing ever more of our attention and awareness, leaving us ever in a state of isolation where screen time is beginning to replace real time.

In a world where there are fake trees, fake bodies, fake people, and fake news, we would think the last place we want this inauthenticity to permeate and bleed into is our most intimate relationships. In an attempt to make reality more real, we will go into our deepest and most intimate relationships first. If we can work on coming out first in these spaces and be accepted for who we are, then we may start to build the confidence to expand that circle of safety outward.

We hide and censor parts of ourselves from our partners, largely because we are afraid that if we reveal our real selves we will be rejected by the person whose love we want the most, whose acceptance we crave the most, and so we continue to go on pretending, censoring, and hiding ourselves, and as we hide one aspect of ourselves we begin to censor other things, other topics of conversation that may lead back to the original topic of censorship, driving an even wider gap between the two until there is so much space between that it can make us seem distant to each other.

So how do we bridge the gap? There are many ways to go about this. Here are merely a few suggestions to help provide an idea of what we are talking about, but also to show how far we can go and that we have been living quite heavily to one side of a line. This is in part to instill and inspire other people to engage with life more boldly, and to not hold back due to our fears and insecurities.

For this we are going to use sex. We go to a therapist and they ask to talk about our childhood, and our response can be something like, "What does that have to do with anything? Let's talk about work, or the game last night." And the therapist perks up at the attempt to redirect the conversation and says, "No, let's talk about your childhood. There was a greater emotional response and a sheer aversion to it, which indicates that there could be something of value if we keep digging." Sex is in the same light as the trigger of asking about someone's childhood. It's a trigger for us, one way or another. Whether it titillates or revolts, it produces strong reactions in us, and much like a trigger point in the body it seems that one of the most simple and straightforward ways to address the tension is through pushing on it. It's not pleasant and can feel counterintuitive, but often afterward the person with the trigger point feels better and has better movement from addressing this issue. Sex acts as a catalyst, stirring the proverbial pot of our hearts and helping us to see what's under the surface. Sex can inspire, move, connect, and separate people in all sorts of ways.

Exercise 1

Grab a paper and pen and sit down alone. Write out your interests, aspirations, hopes, nightmares, taboos, desires, and curiosities, and be as honest as you can here. There is no one else around, and the more honest we can be with ourselves, the more honest we can be with each other. Take note and acknowledge all these parts of ourselves that we often keep hidden from others. Now burn the paper. This is a simple exercise for us to get more acquainted with ourselves, as this is one of the most important relationships we can develop. If we can better understand ourselves and relate to ourselves better, we can understand and connect with other people better as well.

Exercise 2

Have a controversial conversation that is considered a cultural taboo with your partner. An example of this would be asking your partner if they have ever looked at someone else in a desirable way. Often when asked the answer is "no" but the honest truth is that they actually have. You have, they have, and we all have. We know this and yet still continue lying to each other and continue to reinforce ideas of what we think our partner wants to hear. When you inspect our most intimate and deepest relationships, the truth is far more appealing and rewarding.

So, we call each other out on this. Your partner tells you they only have eyes for you. Ok, let's try another way of approaching this. You show your partner something you have never revealed to them before. In this moment, we take the first risk of stepping forward, dropping some of the walls we've put up, revealing a glimpse (often for the first time) of something more real. And having taken the first step toward that risk and dropping some of our defenses, our partners are often moved by the act of our vulnerability; it also shows a little more about themselves that they haven't seen before. For many, this is one of the first times in the relationship where they are being completely honest with each other and no longer work off of a script or routine that brings something real into their lives and relationships.

This act alone can unlock the floodgates, allowing for a tremendous gushing forth of conversation. People quite regularly feel they communicate and talk with their partners, but the truth is when we venture down this path and begin to remove those areas of censorship, we become free to talk about so much more since the metaphorical regulators have been removed.

This practice can cause a lot of insecurities and fears to surface. If we are unwilling to work on these insecurities, it doesn't mean they don't exist. We never had to confront, address, work through, or deal with any of these issues. As mentioned, another catalyst for change is sexual intimacy. How many triggers come up from one simple topic and by that it seems that there are many pearls of wisdom waiting to be gleaned by those brave enough to venture into the hidden worlds inside of us.

These difficult things are similar to strength training: when we move forward instead of shy away from, we grow, become better, and more competent to deal with the trials and tribulations that Life throws at us.

There are many more steps to follow, but these are the first few to get the ball rolling. From here, the next steps are entirely up to you. Whether you leave it there and find solace in your newfound honesty and authenticity, you've got new fertile ground where brand new things will start to sprout, or you can keep going further. Talk is cheap. Actions speak louder than words. There isn't a set protocol as to where to go next or where the end point is because there just isn't one. So where do we go from here? These ideas are only to provide points of gradience from one end of the spectrum to another without a set destination. These are to encourage you to explore the world and our existence with playfulness and curiosity that is authentic so we can discover new unchartered territory where our boundaries get pushed and we can start to redefine our "centre".

For those who have expressed an interest in proceeding, you can begin with a discussion about what that might look like and how you would go about it. You would want to consider what is acceptable and what is off limits. Now that we are going off script to deepen our connections, we need to learn how to be more present, work spontaneously, and enhance our communication skills.

Often for a lot of people who choose to explore open relationships, they start with swinging. It's a start that allows each other to experience a new depth of the relationship in what most would consider operating in safe mode. There is more than one way and certainly no right way or wrong way to this exploration. Some may choose a different relationship structure and explore Polyamory or some form of ethical non-monogamy. Each of our relationships is a snowflake in this journey and you get to choose the open relationship structure that works for you. You can start your research with the many resources online of what is involved and get a general idea of what to expect. Like learning a new recipe, exercise, replacing pavement stones and how to public speak, it's beneficial to educate yourself on this and do more research together after you bring up the conversation with your partner. From there, if you decide on swinging, you can find a lifestyle club where you have date nights so as to experience the atmosphere with others who are either new or experienced in the lifestyle. There are no expectations to be involved, to flirt or engage in anything that you don't want to do. The environment should give you a sense of respect, consent, and lowered inhibitions. It's the cultural motto of a lifestyle club. You and your partner can have drinks, soak in the atmosphere, hit the dance floor, or hang back and observe. The lifestyle clubs provide new and experienced people with the opportunity to tour the facilities and ask any questions they may have. You can meet people anywhere in person and online. Inside the realm of opening up, there are many layers of open that it's up to you to agree upon and explore.

Each layer offers up different challenges that will inspire more communication, inspection, transparency, and more opportunities to grow into a better version of yourself and a better person to your partner. It will test the qualities you define yourself with and it will test you with the certainties you ground yourself and your relationship on. You will welcome a lustful battle within your relationship and most importantly, yourself. These opportunities aren't a way to make superficial relationships that you use and walk away from at the break of dawn, but rather to experience, get messy, and find our Humanity. Unlike other forms of self-development that steer us into personal work on ourselves by making amends for past behaviors, righting our wrongs, or apologize for what we've done, this calls for an extra layer of challenge to invite another along our experimental journey. This too calls for an extension for us and our partner to find others to join this exploration. You ask for a blueprint but there isn't one. The reminder is that mistakes will happen and from those mistakes, there are things we can learn. Like an infant learning to walk, most will fall a lot and from these attempts and undeterred failures, they begin to run. The complexity to which we can grow from falling so many times gives us the understanding that, as we go up this road together, we will make mistakes. The inversion of this scenario is that we stop making mistakes, we stop falling, we become fixed, and we are no longer growing. The process to a handstand involves some falling on our faces at least once or twice and sustaining some injuries like scrapes, bruises, strains and sprains. That is perfectly okay. By stepping into the unknown, we will fail and when we choose to continue, we showcase a message of strength, perseverance, and grit to the younger ones who are observing us every day. We show that we aren't afraid to step up, aren't afraid to step out, aren't afraid to venture into these unknowns and we definitely aren't afraid of mistakes. When we don't, we teach our younger ones to shy away, to not try, and to be afraid of the things we aren't aware or certain of and reinforce the habits that glue them in front of the screen; a screen that won't disappoint, push back, or stimulate and even become scared of the echo of their own voices.

Conclusion

All of this is to set in motion the never-ending journey of self-development. There is no one way to do anything, and it seems if anything we are the spaces between these ideas we see as so fixed. We learn to practice how to stand between two sides and how to embody both masculinity and femininity, how to explore between sitting still and going all the way. This world is so bizarrely immense that there is no end in sight, and when we begin to take interest in one thing, we begin to see how it can lead toward an interest in many things. This shows that things are much bigger than we know, and our reference to our centre is in all likelihood skewed. As we go about pushing against our boundaries and returning to the centre, learning to orchestrate tension and relaxation, how to hold on while letting go, to see the patterns in chaos and to see the work within play and to find play within, our work begins to cultivate a sense of savviness that helps us navigate in the physical, intellectual, and emotional spaces that we occupy.

The suggestions made in this book are there to produce friction, heat, which aids in catalyzing change. Not to say we have to, but when we are open to possibility, we become more open to the possibility that the future can look much brighter. None of this has to be done;

much like working out, you can go through life without challenging yourself physically, as many people have, but it seems if we do expose ourselves to adversity and challenges we are able to grow and do more than we could when we didn't welcome difficulty. Much in the same way we don't have to expose ourselves to different paradigms of the world or see it from different ways, many of us go through our whole lives thinking our thoughts are the only true ones, and that we have the answers compared to everyone else. But when we travel the world or adopt a new perspective, we grow in surprising new ways, and of course this brings us to matters of the heart. You don't have to do what we are proposing in this book, but it seems when we step toward adversity and challenge within our relationships, we tend to become more confident in our competencies to connect, to relate, to understand, and to care. All this is to help us understand better what it means to be ourselves.

www.ingramcontent.com/pod-product-compliance
Lightning Source LLC
LaVergne TN
LVHW011833060526
838200LV00053B/4008